The Tao of Health and Fitness

The Kung-Fu Master's Workout

Jiawen Miao

Multi-Media Books

An imprint of CFW Enterprises, Inc.
Burbank, California

Disclaimer

Please note that the author and publisher of this book are NOT RESPONSIBLE in any manner whatsoever for any injury that may result from practicing the techniques and/or following the instructions given within. Since the physical activities described herein may be too strenuous in nature for some readers to engage in safely, it is essential that a physician be consulted prior to training.

First Published in 2000 by Multi-Media Books, an imprint of CFW Enterprises, Inc.

Library of Congress Catalog Number: 99-76186
ISBN: 1-892515-19-9

Distributed by:
Unique Publications
4201 Vanowen Place
Burbank, CA 91505
(800) 332-3330

Editor: Mark V. Wiley
Cover concept: Stuart Olson
Cover and interior design: Patrick Gross

First Edition
05 04 03 02 01 00 99 98 97 1 3 5 7 9 10 8 6 4 2
Printed in the United States of America

Contents

Introduction 1

PART ONE
BASIC EXERCISE SETS

SET 1. **BREATHING EXERCISES** 7
Lift Up and Press Down 7
Open and Close 9

SET 2. **STRETCHING EXERCISES** 11
Propping Up the Sky 11
Stretching the Chest and Shoulders 12
Swaying Leaves 14
Stretching Side to Side 16
Looking Back 17
Bending Backward and Forward 18
Dragons Entering the Water 20
Looking at Ants 21
Mantis Pose 22

SET 3. **WAIST EXERCISES** 23
Stirring the Waist 23
Floating Boat 25
Pushing Backward 27
Diagonal Stretch 28
Handing in Fruit 30

SET 4. **LEG EXERCISES** 36
Sitting Like a Mountain 36
Squatting Steps 38

Lifting the Body with One Leg 40
Drawing Circles with the Feet 41
Heel Kick 42
Side Kick 43
Laying Legs 44

SET 5.   ARM AND FINGER EXERCISES 46
Pushing Against the Mountain 46
Opening the Door 48
Pulling the Bull's Tail 49
Push Up and Tap 51
Laying Tiger Push-Ups 53

SET 6.   ANKLE EXERCISES 54
Lifting the Heels 54
Popping Up and Down 54

SET 7.   FULL BODY EXERCISES 56
Stretching Like a Cat 56
Looking Around 58
Bull Fighting 60
Weave the Root of a Big Tree 65

SET 8.   RELAXATION EXERCISES 69
Leaves Falling Down 69
Relax by Vibrating 71

SET 9.   DRY BATH EXERCISES 72
Heaven's Drum 72
Face Bath 74
Arm and Leg Bathing 76
Belly Bathing 79

PART TWO
ADVANCED EXERCISE SETS

SET 10. TAI CHI CHUAN EXERCISES 83
Standing Pole 84
Sinking Chi into the Dantian 85
Stepping on Thin Ice 86
Wave Hands Like Fish Tails 90
Drawing a Circle 92
Hanging Leg 96
Pushing Against Waves 98
Waist and Step Turning 99
Working the Millstone 101
Wave Hands Like Clouds 104

SET 11. SINEW TRANSFORMING EXERCISES 107
Preparatory Pose 108
Pressed Palms Pose 109
Extended Arms Pose 110
Propping Up the Sky 111
Catching a Star 113
Pulling the Bull's Tail 115
Forward Push 116
Drawing the Sword 118
Lowering Toward the Ground 120
Extending the Claw 122
Tiger Pose 124
Bang the Drum 126
Pushing Down Pose 127
The Closing Form 128

Introduction

This book provides instruction in traditional Chinese exercises that are designed to promote fitness and good health. The exercises themselves consist of various stationary poses and simple repeated movements. Although at first it may not seem as if these exercises are beneficial, with time you will notice a significant improvement in both your level of fitness and your overall health.

Proper breathing is a fundamental part of these traditional exercises. For this reason, the first exercises presented in this book are designed to help you learn how to breathe in the correct manner. With proper breathing, you fill your body with good oxygen and expel unwanted waste material. This is vital for maintaining good health. Correct breathing techniques also promote the flow of *chi*. *Chi* is a vital energy that our bodies depend upon for health and longevity.

Following the breathing exercises, this book will teach you methods for improving your flexibility and ease of movement. Finally, you will learn exercises designed to strengthen and tone your muscles and tendons.

Many of the exercises in this book are over a thousand years old. They have been handed down and improved upon by generations of martial arts masters. Many of the masters living in China and elsewhere today are living proof of the benefits of these traditional exercises. Although these masters are advanced in age and perhaps do not appear particularly young, their bodies and minds are still youthful and healthy.

As a general rule, when performing these exercises, remain focused on each movement rather than allowing yourself to daydream. Concentrate on keeping your breathing rhythmic and in harmony with your movements. Your body movements should be slow, soft, and graceful. Remain alert. Concentrate your spirit inwardly while appearing peaceful outwardly.

These exercises are designed to promote internal and external health and fitness. When we speak of internal health, we are referring to the cultivation and circulation of vital energy, or *chi*. External health refers to the toning and strengthening of muscles, bones, tendons, and ligaments.

These exercises can be adjusted to your specific needs. In the beginning, just do as many repetitions as feels comfortable for you. Later, increase the number of repetitions for each exercise.

Not much flexibility is needed for these exercises. But, as you progress in your study, you will notice an improvement in your flexibility.

In order to gain any benefits from these exercises, you must practice them on a regular schedule. We suggest at least three times a week. And if all these exercises are performed, your entire body will benefit.

Although these exercises were developed by martial artists, most of them are simple enough for a person with no martial arts experience to learn. If some of the exercises are too difficult for you, just skip them for now. Later, as your skills and fitness improve, you can go back to the more difficult ones.

You do not have to go through all the exercises each time you practice. The quality of your practice is more important than the number of exercises you perform each time. In other words, perform each exercise with care and accuracy, and just pick a few of your favorite exercises from each category.

Although some of the exercises emphasize a particular part of the body, you should concentrate on coordinating your entire body with each movement. Part of the purpose of these exercises is to harmonize your movement, breathing, and mind.

When practicing these exercises, adhere to the following:

- Practice in a quiet location that has a supply of fresh air, but not a place that is excessively windy.

- Before practice, be sure to go to the bathroom. Wear loose clothing. Do not drink too much water.

- After practice, avoid cold or windy places.

- Do not practice right after a meal or when you feel excessively tired.

- If you feel ill after practice, it is probably because you were too tense during the exercises.

PART ONE
BASIC EXERCISE SETS

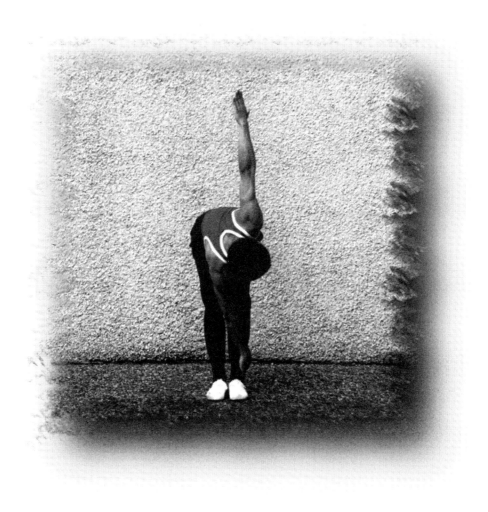

SET 1
BREATHING EXERCISES

Proper breathing is fundamental to all health and fitness exercises. A correct breathing pattern helps you to coordinate and control your body movement. It also promotes peace of mind and concentration. Correct breathing also supplies your body with good oxygen and expels unwanted wastes.

Breathe calmly and deeply while performing these exercises. After inhaling, pause for a moment before exhaling. Do not switch suddenly from an inhale to an exhale or vise-versa. Contract your abdomen when inhaling and expand your abdomen when exhaling. You will feel the vital energy, or *chi*, gather in your abdomen when you breathe in this manner.

Stand in a relaxed posture with your feet parallel and a shoulders-width apart. Keep your head up and your shoulders relaxed. Keep your spine straight. Allow your fingers to be open and relaxed. They may bend inward a little. Look forward. Keep your mouth closed and allow your tongue to rest with its tip touching the roof of your mouth just behind your front teeth.

Lift Up and Press Down
Inhale while lifting your palms from your abdomen to chest level (Figs. 1, 2). Exhale while lowering your palms from your chest to abdomen level (Figs. 3, 4). Breathe deeply and slowly. Do not tense your shoulders while raising your hands. Repeat two to 12 times.

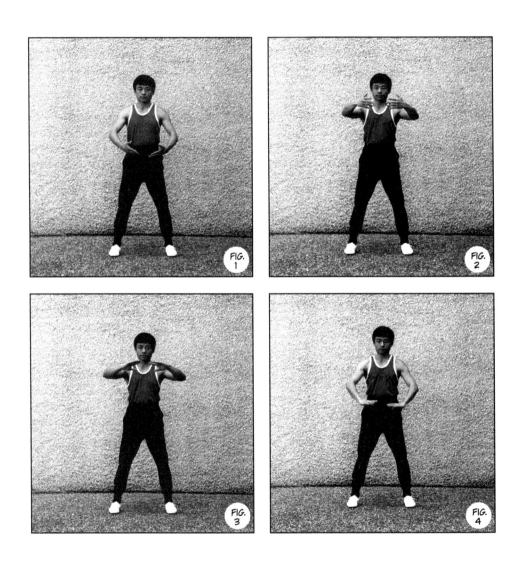

Open and Close

Imagine that you are standing in a pool of warm water with the water up to the level of your shoulders. Begin the exercise with your hands in front of you as if they were holding a small balloon (Fig. 5). As you inhale, spread your hands apart (Fig. 6). Allow your hands to bend inward slightly as if they were encountering resistance from the pool of water in which you are standing. Keep your shoulders relaxed.

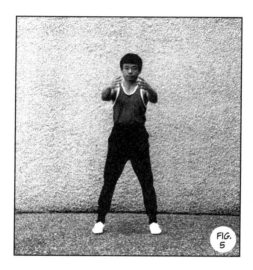

FIG. 5

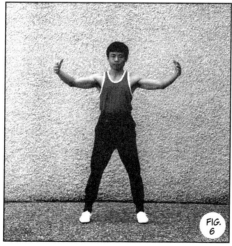

FIG. 6

As you exhale, bring your hands together (Figs. 7, 8). Again, imagine that there is resistance from the water you are standing in. Allow your hands to bend outward slightly as they come together. Repeat the exercise three to 12 times.

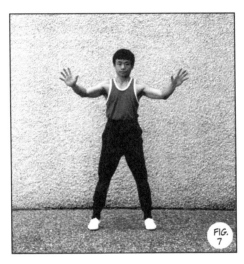

FIG. 7

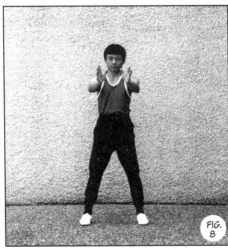

FIG. 8

SET 2
STRETCHING EXERCISES

These stretching exercises have two purposes. The first is to stretch your tendons and muscles so as to promote relaxation. The second is to prepare your body for the more strenuous exercises in the following sections.

Repeat each exercise several times.

Propping Up the Sky

Stand up straight. Lift your hands from the level of your abdomen with your palms facing upward and your fingers pointing toward the center of your body (Fig. 1). As your hands reach the level of your head, turn your palms toward your face (Fig. 2).

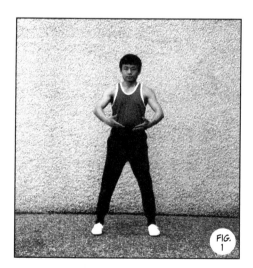
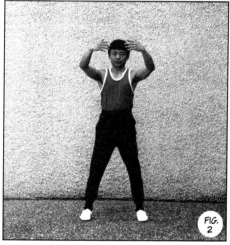

FIG. 1

FIG. 2

As your hands pass the top of your head, turn your palms toward the sky. Then stretch upward as high as you can (Fig. 3). Pretend you are pressing against the sky. Now relax as you lower your hands to your sides (Fig. 4). Inhale as you lift your hands up and exhale as you lower your hands.

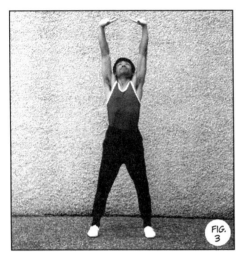

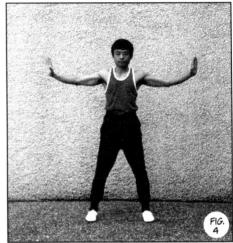

Stretching the Chest and Shoulders

Bend your arms and lift your elbows to shoulder level, with your palms facing downward (Fig. 5). Draw your elbows backward while inhaling to stretch the muscles in your chest (Fig. 6). Then slowly exhale as you reach forward with your hands (Fig. 7). Now rotate your hands until your palms face upward and swing your outstretched arms backward until you feel the muscles in your chest begin to stretch, inhaling as you do so (Fig. 8). Finally, relax and exhale as you bring your arms toward the center of your body, then down toward your abdomen.

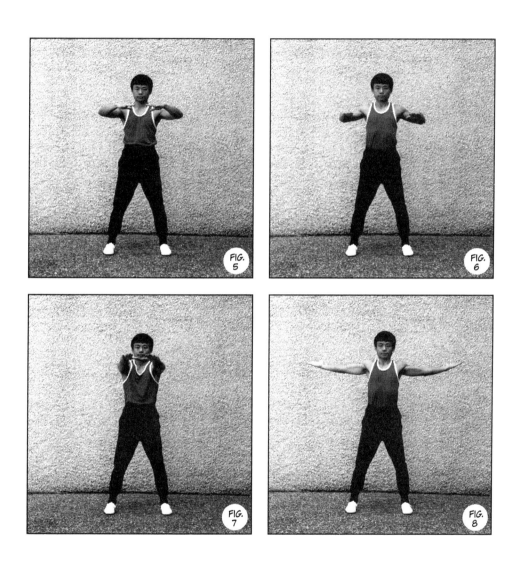

Swaying Leaves

Extend both arms forward with the left hand on top and both palms facing downward (Fig. 9). Turn your body to the left, spread your arms, and turn your palms to face upward (Fig. 10). Keep turning to the left until your torso is facing as far to the left as possible. Your arms should be aligned, with your left arm stretched behind you. Your head should be rotated so that your are facing your left arm. Hold this posture for a moment (Fig. 11). Inhale as you rotate your body. Now exhale and turn back to face front. Allow your arms to stretch to the front with your right hand on top (Fig. 12). Now turn to the right in a mirror image of your left turn, inhaling as you do so (Figs. 13, 14). Exhale as you turn back to face front.

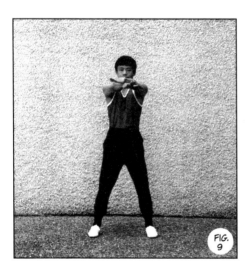

FIG. 9

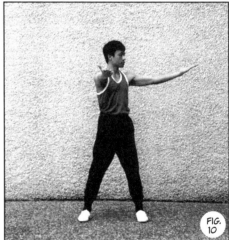

FIG. 10

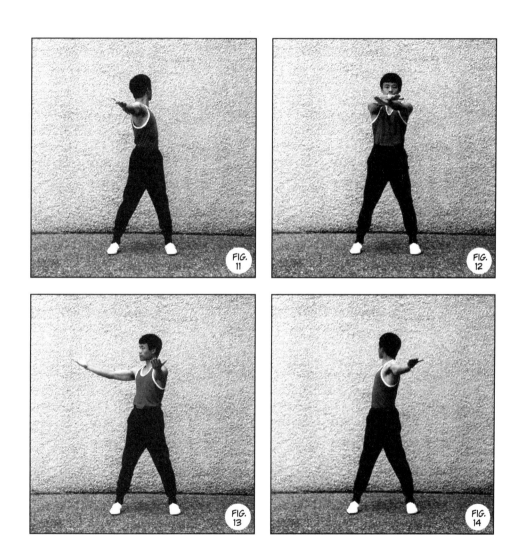

Stretching Side to Side

Spread your arms to the left and right side (Fig. 15). Lift your left arm over the top of your head. Allow your right arm to rest in a relaxed position with your right hand on your hip. Bend your body to the right with your left palm facing downward (Fig. 16). Inhale as you bend to the side. Hold this pose briefly. Now, return to the starting position, exhaling as you do so (Fig. 17). Repeat to the left side (Fig. 18).

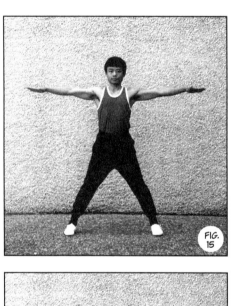

FIG. 15

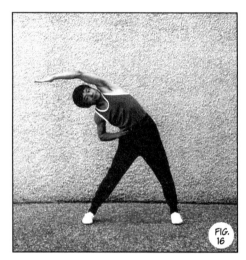

FIG. 16

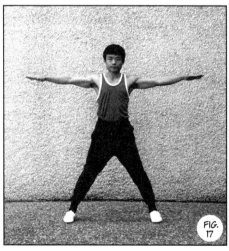

FIG. 17

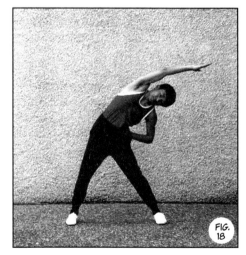

FIG. 18

Looking Back

Stand straight with your hands hanging down to either side. Lift both hands with the palms facing upward to your abdomen, inhaling as you do so (Fig. 19). Then press your hands downward to either side as you turn your head to look back and to the left (Fig. 20). Turn back to the center and relax your arms as you exhale (Fig. 21). Now repeat this motion to the right side (Fig. 22).

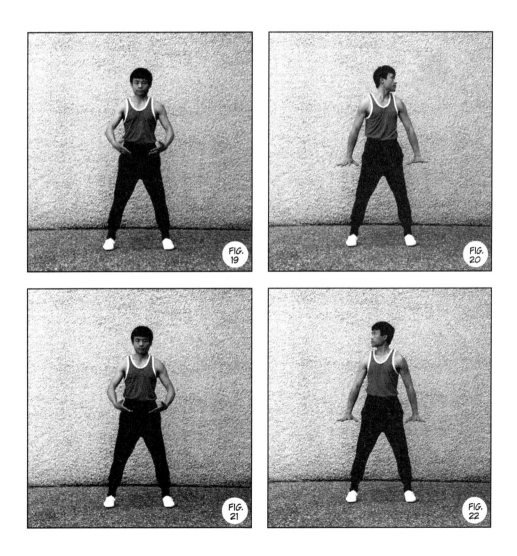

FIG. 19

FIG. 20

FIG. 21

FIG. 22

Bending Backward and Forward

Stand in a relaxed posture with both fists resting on your lower back (Fig. 23). Inhale while bending backward (Fig. 24).

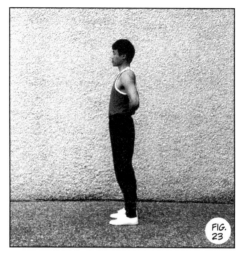

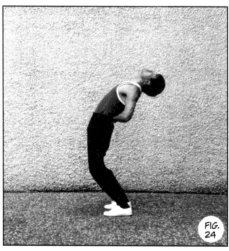

Now exhale as you bend forward (Fig. 25). Allow your hands to slide down the back of your leg as you bend forward (Fig. 26). Raise your body up again, allowing your hands to slide along the inside of your thighs (Fig. 27). Inhale as you rise. When you reach an upright position, allow your hands to rest in a relaxed position at your sides (Fig. 28).

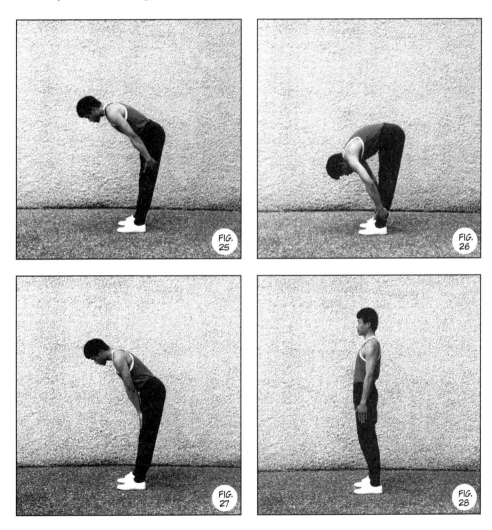

Dragons Entering the Water

Stand with your feet together. Draw your elbows back until your palms are alongside your chest, inhaling as you do so (Fig. 29). Stretch your arms forward as you sink down into a squat, exhaling as you do so. As you reach a full squat, your arms should be stretched forward as far as possible (Figs. 30, 31).

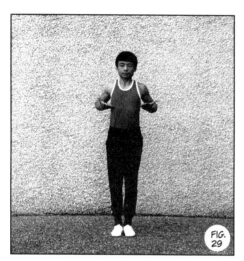

FIG. 29

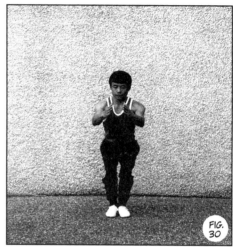

FIG. 30

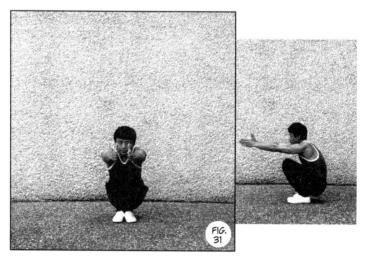

FIG. 31

Looking at Ants

Extend your right leg to the side with the heel of your foot touching the ground. Lift your hands to chest level as you inhale (Fig. 32). Bend down and reach for your toe with your hands, exhaling as you do so (Fig. 33). Repeat to the opposite side (Figs. 34, 35).

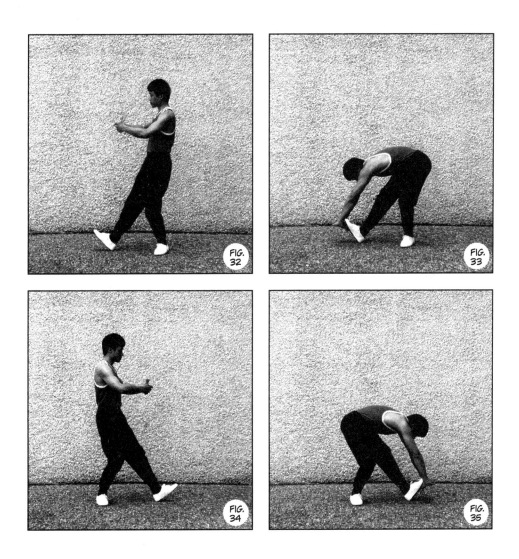

Mantis Pose

Turn your torso to the right and step forward with your right leg. Extend your arms in front of your torso with the palms of your hands facing inward and your fingers interlocked (Fig. 36) As you inhale, push upward with your hands, palms outward, and bend down on your left knee (Fig. 37). Relax and stand up as you exhale. Repeat to the opposite side (Figs. 38, 39).

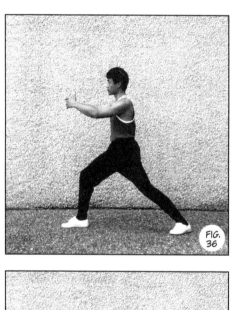

FIG. 36

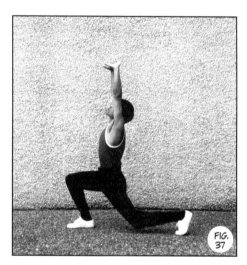

FIG. 37

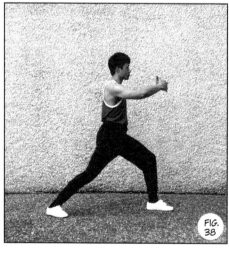

FIG. 38

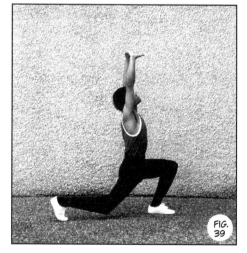

FIG. 39

SET 3
WAIST EXERCISES

An old Chinese saying maintains that the waist ages more rapidly than other parts of the body. Unfortunately, as any athlete or dancer knows, the waist and legs are to the body like the foundation of a house—without a strong foundation, a house will sooner or later crumble to the ground. For this reason, the ancient Chinese placed a great deal of importance on maintaining strength and mobility in the waist.

Stirring the Waist

Make a circular motion with your waist, as if using a hoola hoop. As your waist circles to the right, lean your torso to the left (Fig. 1) As your waist circles to the rear, lean forward (Fig. 2) and as your waist circles to the left, lean your torso to the right (Fig. 3). Finally, lean backward as your waist circles to the front (Fig. 4).

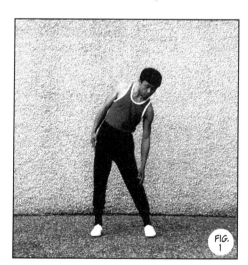
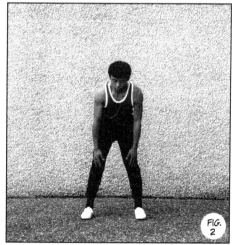

FIG. 1

FIG. 2

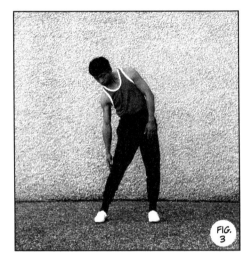

FIG.
3

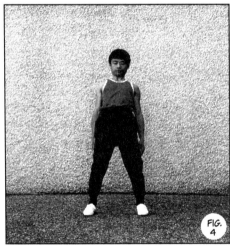

FIG.
4

Floating Boat

Bend your knees and relax your body (Fig. 5). Turn your body to the left, straighten your legs a little, and lift both arms so that they are in a straight line with one another (Fig. 6). Look to your left as you do so (Fig. 7). Then lower your arms, bend your knees a little, and turn back to face forward.

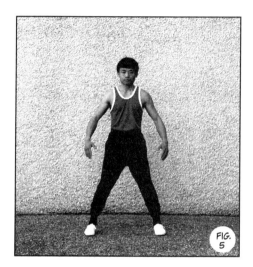
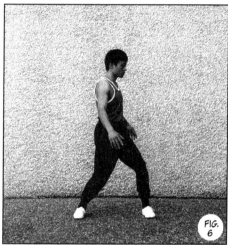

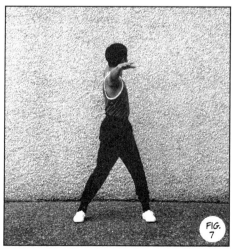

Repeat to the opposite side (Figs. 8–10). This exercise should be performed in a relaxed manner with your arms swinging back and forth in a flowing, gentle movement.

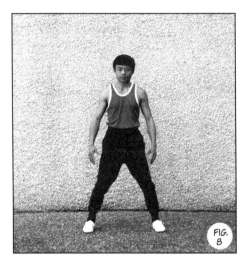

FIG.
8

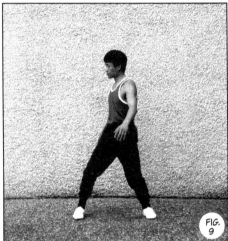

FIG.
9

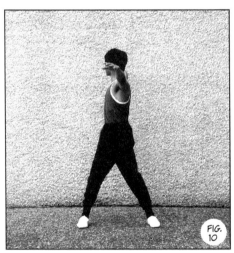

FIG.
10

Pushing Backward

Bend your knees as if riding on a horse. Keep your torso erect and your hands, closed into fists, at your waist (Fig. 11). Turn to the right, and push your left arm across your torso and past your right shoulder with your fingers outspread (Fig. 12). Turn to the front and draw your left hand to your waist again (Fig. 13). Repeat to the opposite side (Fig. 14).

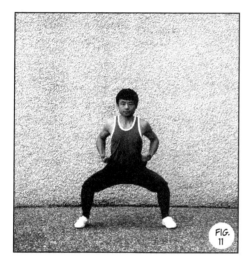
FIG. 11

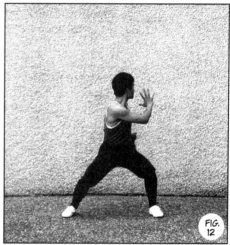
FIG. 12

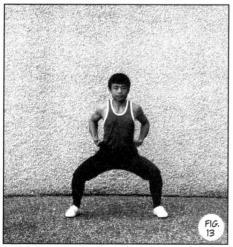
FIG. 13

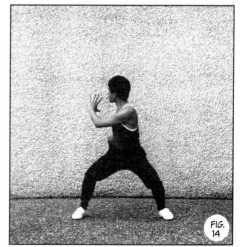
FIG. 14

Diagonal Stretch

In a relaxed standing position, raise your right arm up and to the right (Fig. 15). Now swing your arm down across your body to the lower left, reaching for your left toe (Fig. 16). Swing your left arm up and behind you (Fig. 17). Repeat to the opposite side (Figs. 18–20).

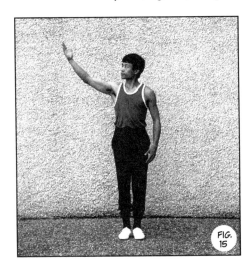

FIG. 15

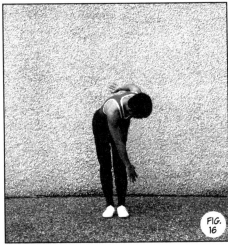

FIG. 16

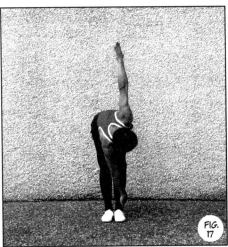

FIG. 17

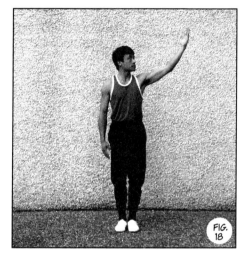

FIG.
18

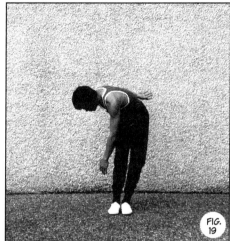

FIG.
19

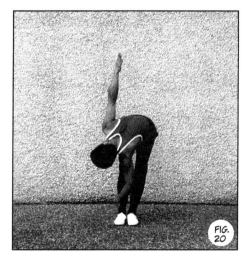

FIG.
20

Handing in Fruit

Imaging that you are holding a bowl of water in either hand (Fig. 21). Turn to the left and swing your right hand, palm upward, to your navel (Fig. 22). Rotate your right hand in a counter-clockwise motion so that the fingers point to the right side (Fig. 23). Now push your right hand in an upward arc, rotating your wrist as you do so, up over your head and to the left side (Fig. 24).

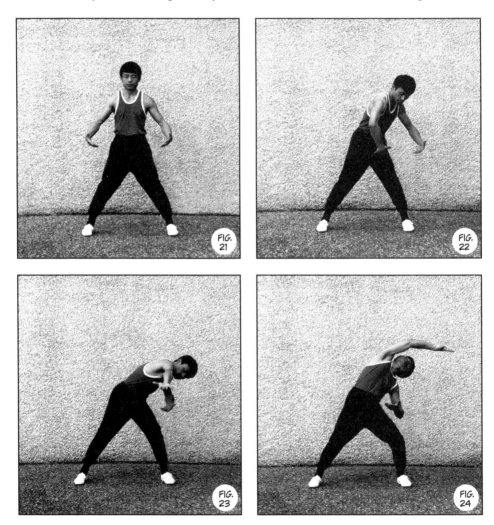

FIG. 21

FIG. 22

FIG. 23

FIG. 24

Swing your right hand behind and to the right (Fig. 25). Continue to swing your right hand to the right, leaning in that direction as you do so (Fig. 26). Now swing your right hand to the center of your body and draw your right hand in toward your abdomen as you stretch your left hand forward (Fig. 27). Stretch your left arm to the left side (Fig. 28).

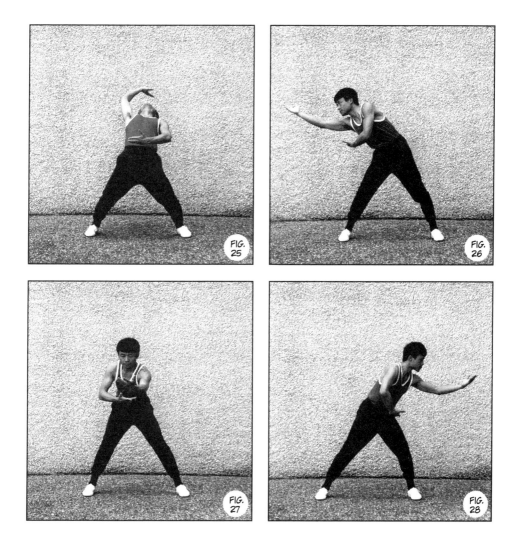

In the following sequence you will be rotating your body counterclockwise. Begin by bending backward as you simultaneously twist your right hand, drawing a circle in front of your navel, while reaching overhead with your left arm, palm up (Fig. 29). As your body reaches the right, and you are facing front again, your right hand should have rotated again, leaving it palm up, as you reach overhead to the right with your left arm (Fig. 30). Continue the circle by bending forward and reaching your left arm toward the left (Fig. 31) and around you to your back (Fig. 32).

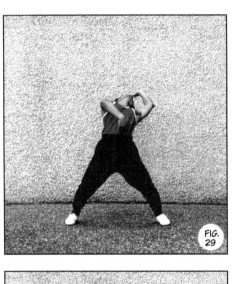

FIG. 29

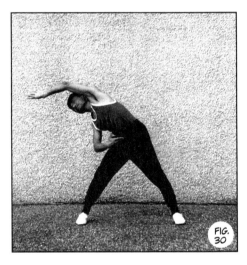

FIG. 30

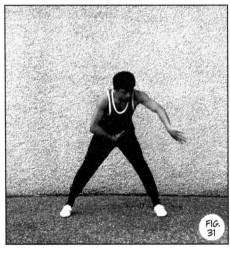

FIG. 31

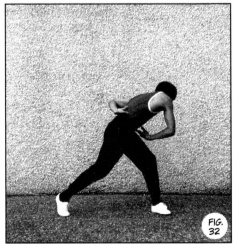

FIG. 32

Twist your torso to the front again as you extend your left arm to the left (Fig. 33) and then over your head to the right as you straighten (Fig. 34). Bend backward again to the left, ending up facing right with your left hand held head level and your right hand held navel level, both palms facing you (Figs. 35, 36).

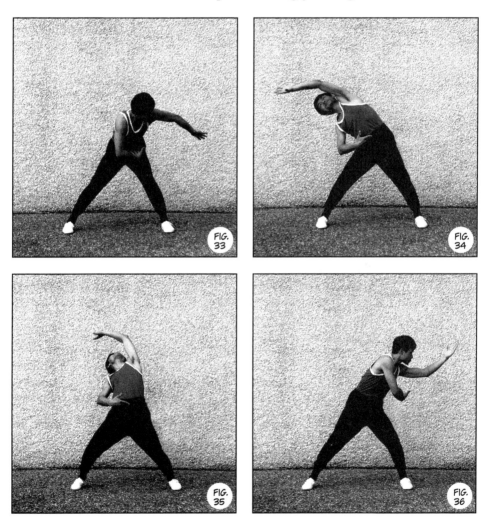

FIG. 33

FIG. 34

FIG. 35

FIG. 36

From here, face the front again and switch hand positions (Fig. 37). Repeat the core movements of the above sequence, this time with the right hand (Figs. 38–42).

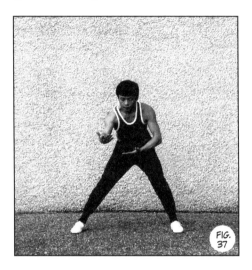

When doing this exercise, your eyes should follow your hands, your body is stirring with your waist as the axis, and your palms always face upward. Inhale while bending forward and exhale while bending backward.

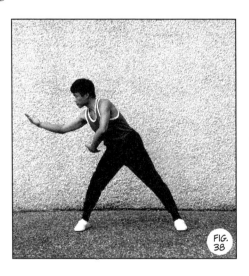

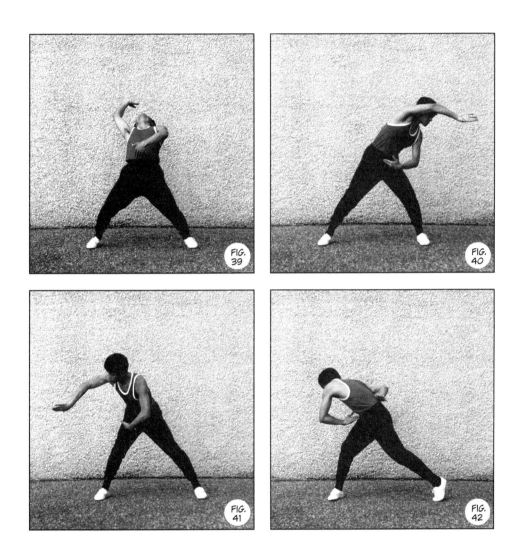

FIG.
39

FIG.
40

FIG.
41

FIG.
42

SET 4
LEG EXERCISES

Sitting Like a Mountain

Stand with your legs at shoulder width. Raise your hands up to shoulder level with your palms facing upward (Fig. 1). Turn your palms downward and sink slowly into a squat until your thighs are parallel to the ground (Figs. 2, 3).

When squatting, keep your torso erect. Inhale as you rise up and exhale as you squat down.

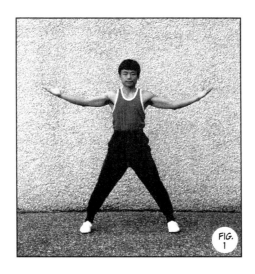

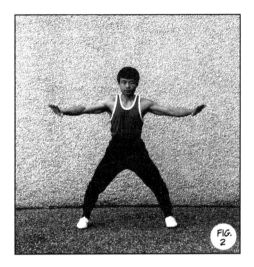

FIG. 2

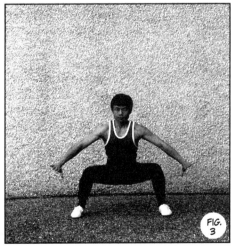

FIG. 3

Squatting Steps

Stand with your legs wider than shoulder width. Allow your arms to rest parallel to the ground in a relaxed position (Fig. 4). Shift your weight to the right and bend your right knee (Fig. 5). Keep your left leg straight and sink down as low as possible (Fig. 6). Keep both feet flat on the ground. Repeat to the opposite side (Figs. 7–9). Inhale as you rise up and exhale as you sink down.

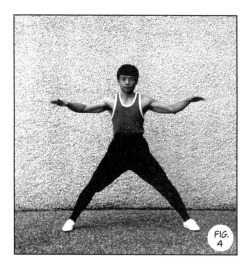

FIG. 4

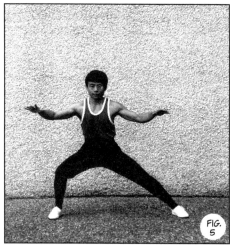

FIG. 5

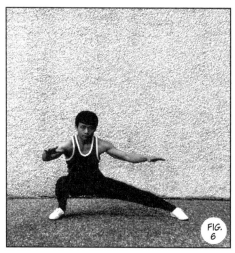

FIG. 6

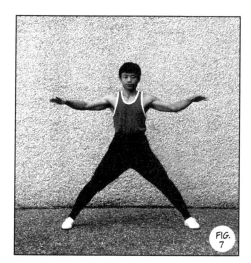

FIG. 7

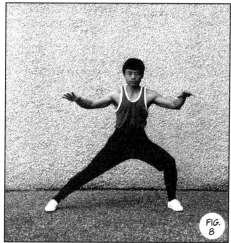

FIG. 8

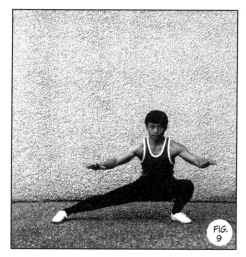

FIG. 9

Lifting the Body with One Leg

Stand on one leg while lifting the other leg to horizontal level (Fig. 10). Bend the standing leg and slowly sink down, keeping the other leg horizontal (Fig. 11). Now rise up on the bent leg (Fig. 12). Repeat several times then switch legs and do the same thing on the opposite side. *Please note that this is an advanced exercise.* Do NOT attempt this until your legs are strong enough to support your body in this manner.

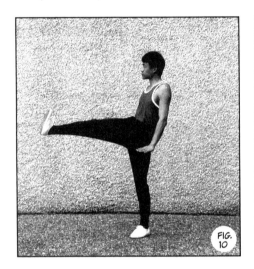

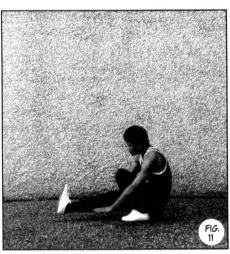

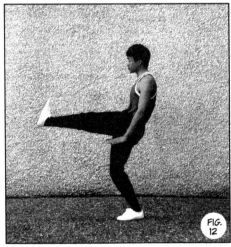

Drawing Circles with the Feet

Stand on your left leg with your hands out to either side (Fig. 13). Allow your right leg to hang with the knee bent. Draw a circle in the air with your right foot to loosen up your right knee (Figs. 14–16). Rotate your arms slightly as you do so to help retain your balance. Repeat to the opposite side.

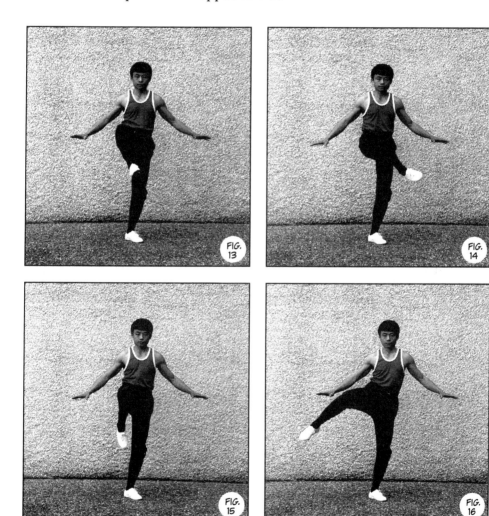

FIG. 13

FIG. 14

FIG. 15

FIG. 16

Heel Kick

Stand on your left leg and chamber your right leg with the right knee bent. Extend your two hands to your sides with your palms facing downward to help maintain your balance (Fig. 17). Kick forward with your toes pointed back and your heel out (Fig. 18). Kick several times, then switch to the other leg.

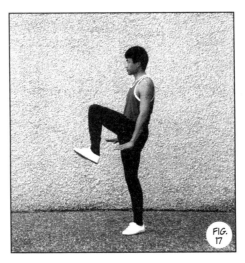

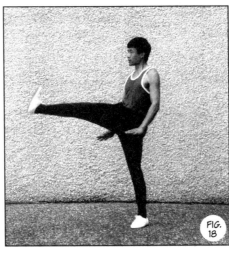

Side Kick

Stand on your left leg and chamber your right leg with the right knee bent. Place your two hands at your sides with your palms facing downward to help maintain your balance (Fig. 19). Kick to the side with your foot angled toward the center of your body (Fig. 20). Kick several times, then switch to the other leg.

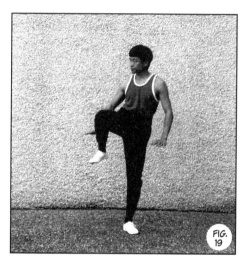

FIG. 19

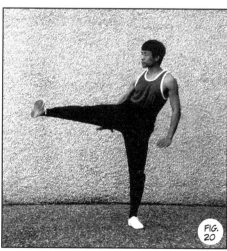

FIG. 20

Laying Legs

Stand with your legs beyond shoulder width. Lift your hands to chest level (Fig. 21). Shift your weight to the left and squat down on your left leg (Fig. 22). Keep your left foot flat on the ground and rest your right foot on its heel (Fig. 23). Stand up slowly (Fig. 24).

Be sure to exhale while squatting and to inhale while rising up.

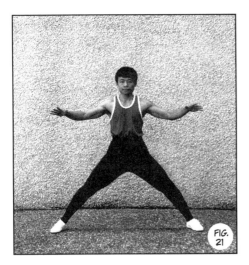
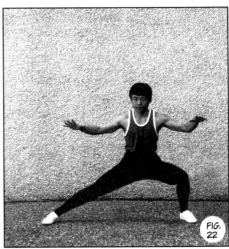
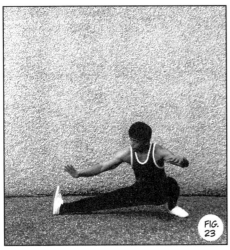
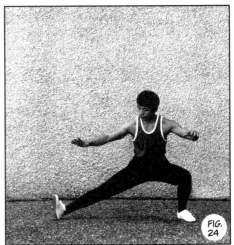

Repeat to the opposite side (Figs. 25–28)

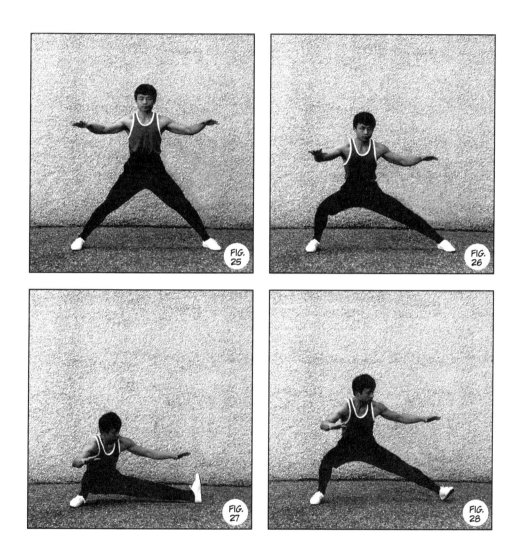

SET 5
ARM AND FINGER EXERCISES

Pushing Against the Mountain

Stand with your feet slightly beyond shoulder width. Lift your hands up to shoulder level as you inhale (Fig. 1). Sink down into a squat (Fig. 2). As you sink down, push your hands toward the center of your body and forward (Figs. 3, 4). Exhale as you push your hands forward.

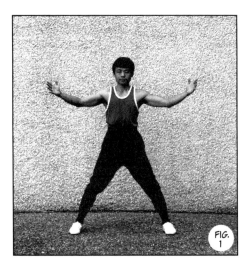

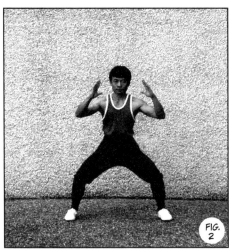

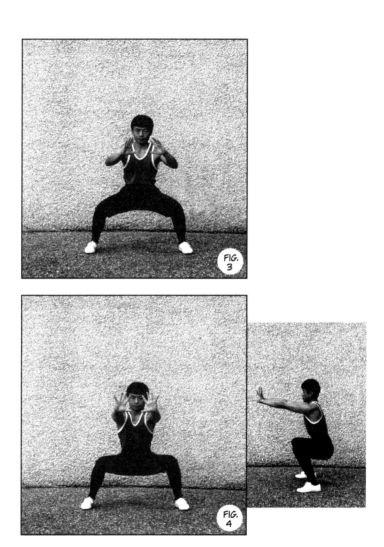

FIG.
3

FIG.
4

Opening the Door

Stand with your feet slightly beyond shoulder width and your legs slightly bent. Lift your hands up to shoulder level with palms facing inward as you inhale (Fig. 5). Bend your elbows and push your palms to either side (Fig. 6). Then squat down, exhale, and stretch your arms out to either side with your palms facing outward (Fig. 7).

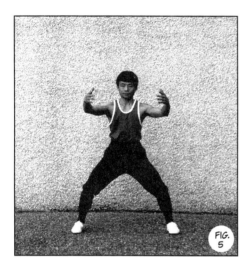

FIG. 5

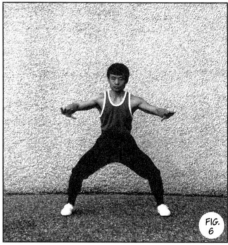

FIG. 6

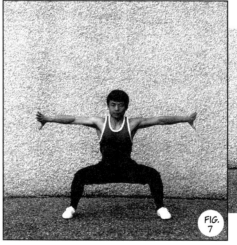

FIG. 7

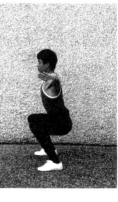

Pulling the Bull's Tail

Extend your right leg to the right side. Curl your right arm with your hand in a fist. Hold your left arm behind you with the hand in a fist (Fig. 8). Imagine pulling a weight backward with your right arm, bending backward and exhaling as you do so (Fig. 9). Now pull with your left arm and lean forward (Fig. 10).

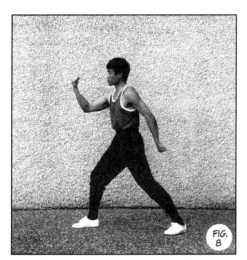

FIG. 8

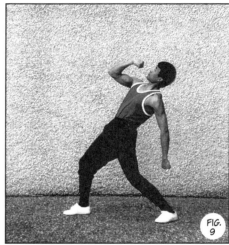

FIG. 9

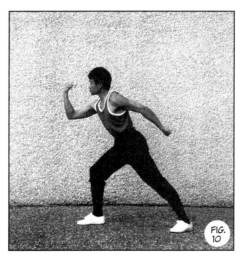

FIG. 10

Repeat to the left side (Figs. 11–13).

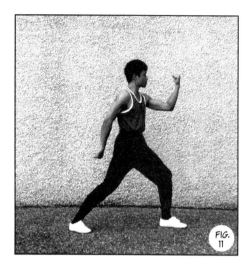

FIG.
11

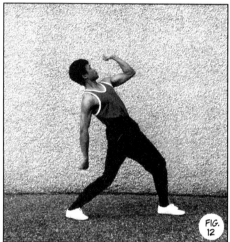

FIG.
12

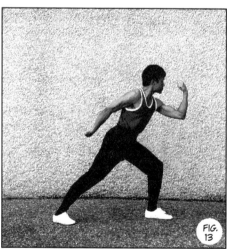

FIG.
13

Push Up and Tap

Start in a regular push-up posture, with legs extended and arms locked elevating the upper body (Fig. 14). Bend your elbows to lower your chest to the ground (Fig. 15). Inhale as you do this.

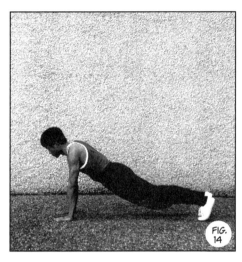

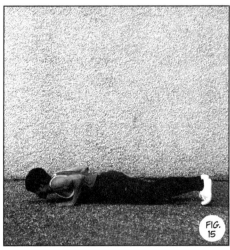

Exhale as you push your body up. Upon reaching full arm extension, clap your hands together (Fig. 16), landing on your fingertips (Fig. 17). After a moment, allow your palms to drop back down to the floor so that they support your weight once again, and perform another push up in this manner (Fig. 18). Repeat.

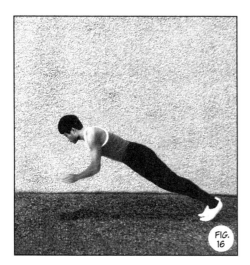

FIG. 16

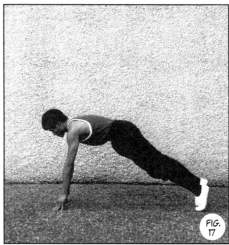

FIG. 17

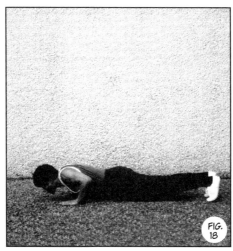

FIG. 18

Laying Tiger Push-Ups

Step into a lunge position with your right leg in front. Bend down and support part of your weight with your fingers (Fig. 19). Lower your body by bending your right knee and both elbows while exhaling (Fig. 20). Push up while inhaling.

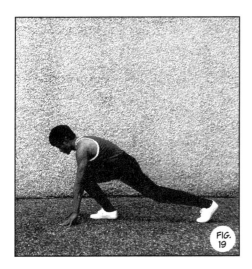
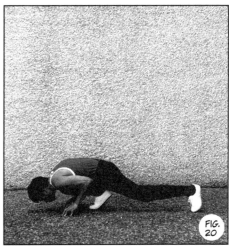

Repeat to the opposite side (Figs. 21, 22).

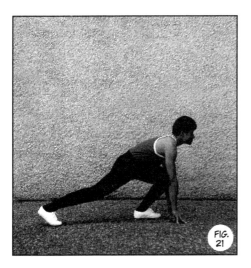
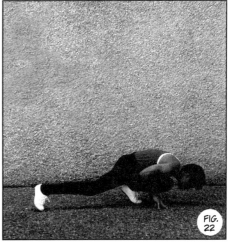

Set 6
ANKLE EXERCISES

Lifting the Heels

Stand naturally with your feet together (Fig. 1). Lift your heels off the ground slowly as you inhale (Fig. 2). Pause for a moment, then lower your heels to the ground slowly as you exhale.

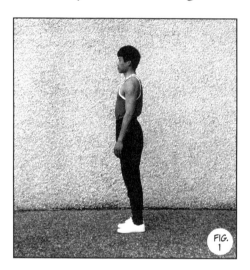 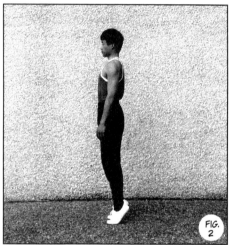

Popping Up and Down

Stand with your feet at shoulder width. Lift your hands to shoulder level with your palms facing upward (Fig. 3). Now drop your hands, with palms facing downward, toward the ground as you simultaneously sink down into a squat (Fig. 4). Unlike the previous squats, however, lift your heels off the ground as you sink down (Fig. 5). Exhale as you sink down. Turn your palms so that they are facing upward as you rise up (Fig. 6). Inhale as you rise.

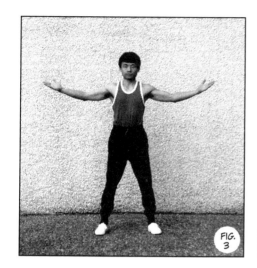

FIG.
3

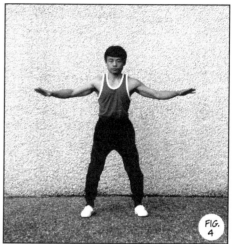

FIG.
4

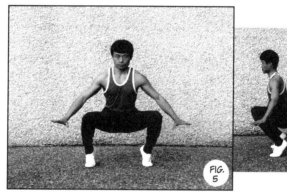

FIG.
5

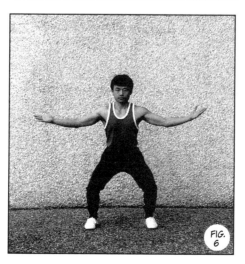

FIG.
6

Set 7
FULL BODY EXERCISES

Stretching Like a Cat

Begin in a posture similar to that when beginning a push-up, but with your hands slightly closer to your waist (Fig. 1). Push your body up and back, stretching your arms and shoulders and inhaling as you do so (Fig. 2). Now bend your elbows and lower your body toward the ground as you exhale (Fig. 3). Push your torso forward and then up to the original position (Figs. 4, 5).

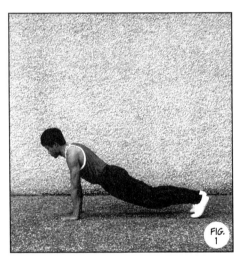

FIG. 1

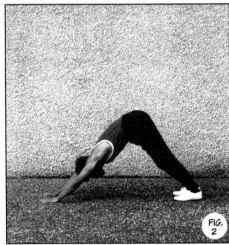

FIG. 2

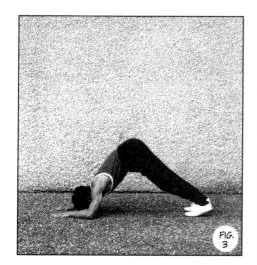

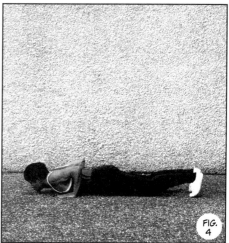

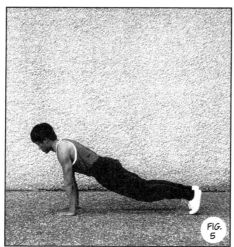

Looking Around

Stand with your feet slightly beyond shoulder width and your arms up at chest level (Fig. 6). Turn your waist and head to the right (Fig. 7). As you turn your torso and head fully to the right, stretch your left arm up and your right arm down toward your left heel (Fig. 8). Inhale as you twist. Turn back to the center, exhaling as you do so (Fig. 9). Repeat the exercise to the opposite side (Figs. 10, 11).

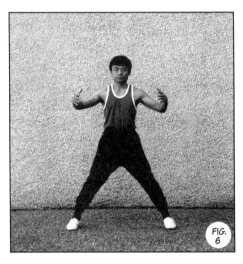

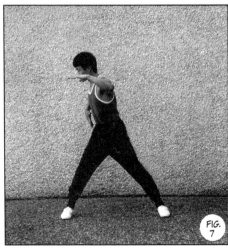

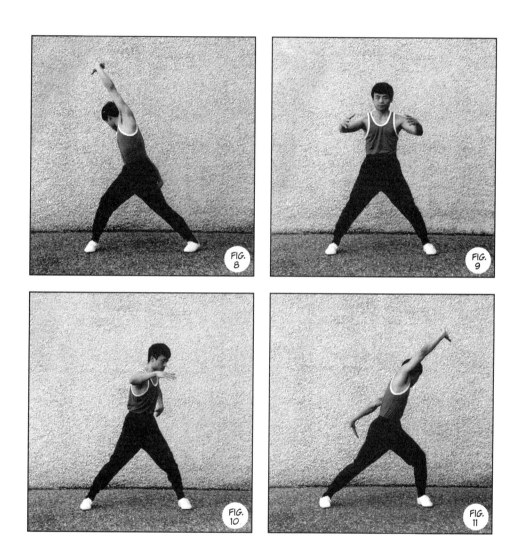

FIG. 8

FIG. 9

FIG. 10

FIG. 11

Bull Fighting

Stand with your feet a double shoulders-width apart, knees bent, extending and holding your arms out to their respective sides (Fig. 12). Shift your weight onto your left leg (Fig. 13). Turn your torso to the right and extend your left arm toward the front (Fig. 14). Shift your weight onto your right leg as you rotate your torso to the right and extend your left arm forward (Fig. 15).

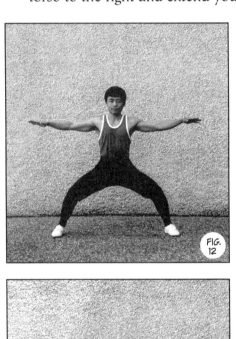
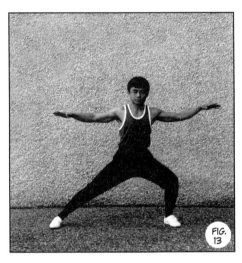
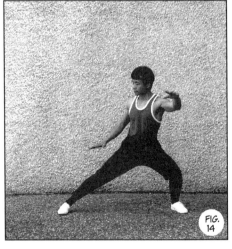
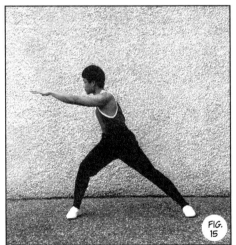

Sink down lower on your right leg and turn your torso to the left, so that you are now facing forward. While turning, reach out with your right arm and lower your left arm (Fig. 16). Shift your weight onto your left leg and reach to the left with your right arm (Fig. 17). Then reach with your left arm while lowering your right arm (Fig. 18). Turn your torso to the right (Fig. 19).

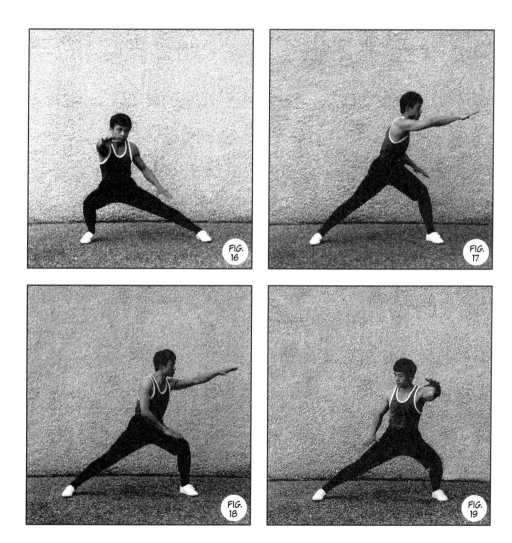

FIG. 16

FIG. 17

FIG. 18

FIG. 19

Shift your weight forward onto your right foot as you reach forward with your left arm (Fig. 20). Extend your right arm and lower your left arm (Fig. 21). Turn your torso to the front (Fig. 22). Shift your weight onto your left leg and extend your right arm forward (Fig. 23).

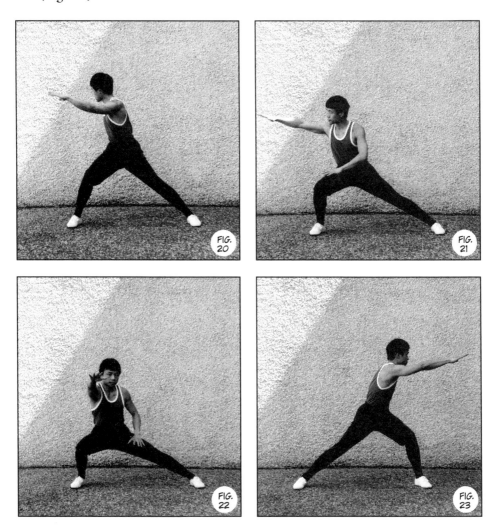

FIG. 20

FIG. 21

FIG. 22

FIG. 23

Lower your right arm as you reach forward with your left arm (Fig. 24). Extend your right arm forward (Fig. 25). Now shift your weight onto your right leg and extend your right arm forward (Fig. 26). Turn your torso to the left, keeping your right arm extended (Fig. 27).

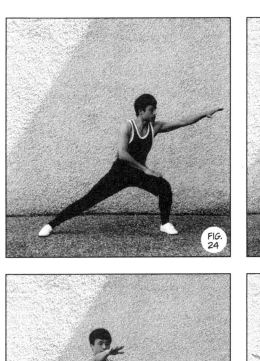

FIG. 24

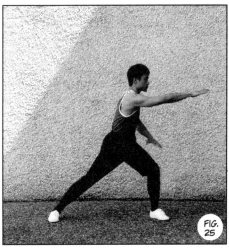

FIG. 25

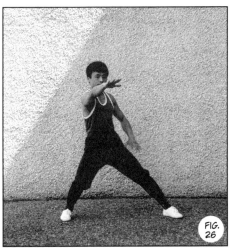

FIG. 26

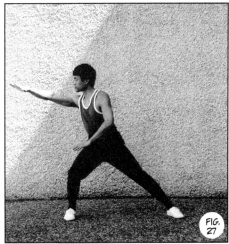

FIG. 27

Keep turning your torso so that you are looking behind you (Fig. 28). Now turn your torso to the left, with your left arm extended forward (Fig. 29). Turn your torso completely to the left, stretching forward with your left arm (Fig. 30.) Continue to shift to the left and the right while waving your arms back and forth.

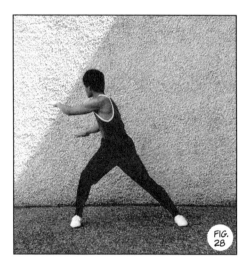

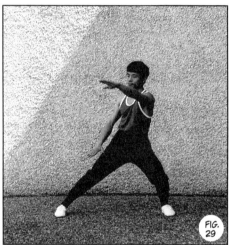

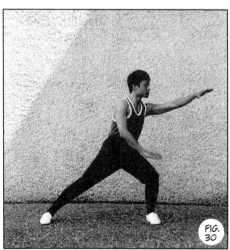

Weave the Root of a Big Tree

Stand with your feet at shoulders-width. Raise your hands to chest level with your elbows bent, palms facing your chest (Fig. 31). Turn to the right while placing your right hand behind your back and your left hand in front of your chest (Fig. 32). Continue to turn all the way around, allowing your legs to cross as you do so (Fig. 33). Continue turning all the way around and stretch your right arm to your rear as you sink down onto your left knee (Fig. 34).

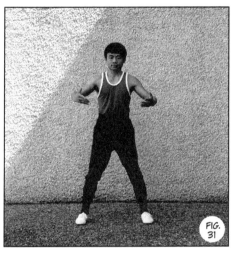

FIG. 31

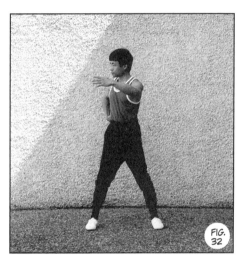

FIG. 32

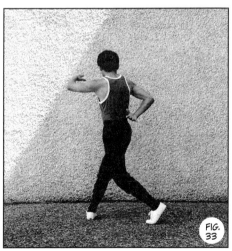

FIG. 33

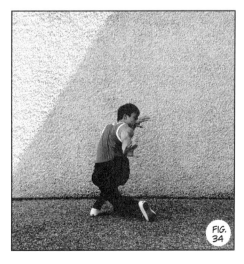

FIG. 34

Turn back to center in the following manner—keeping the right arm extended (Figs. 35–37).

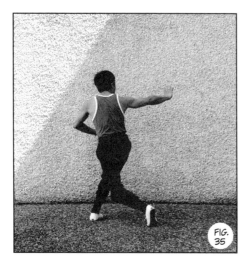

FIG. 35

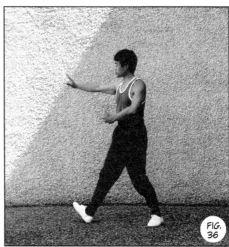

FIG. 36

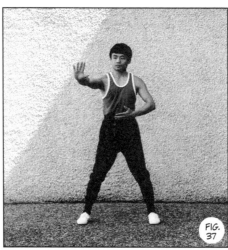

FIG. 37

Repeat to the opposite side—this time extending the left arm to the rear (Figs. 38–40).

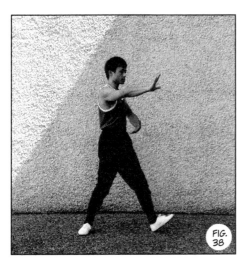

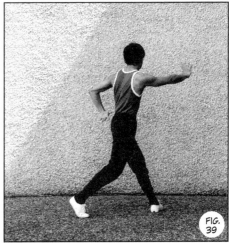

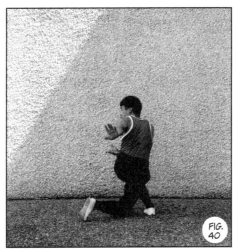

Turn back to center—keeping the left arm extended (Figs. 41–43)—and switch to the other side again.

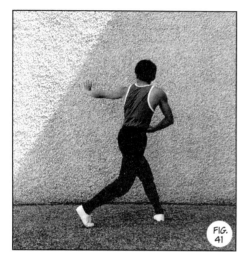

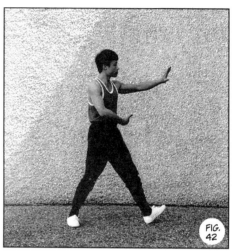

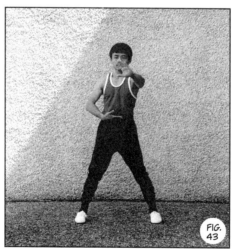

SET 8
RELAXATION EXERCISES

Leaves Falling Down

Begin with your feet a shoulders-width apart and arms at your sides. Lift your arms slowly, palms facing in (Fig. 1). Continue to lift your arms, turning your palms to face upward as your hands pass above your shoulders (Fig. 2). Allow your arms to reach their maximum extension above your head, then turn your palms inward (Fig. 3).

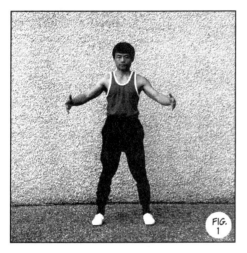

FIG. 1

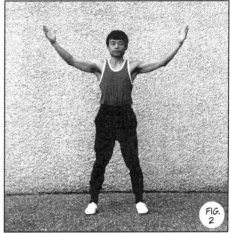

FIG. 2

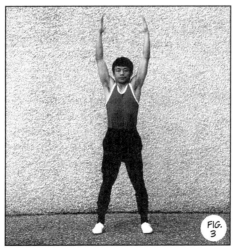

FIG. 3

Now, with your palms facing downward, lower your hands over your head and down to the front of your body in one smooth motion (Figs. 4, 5). Finally, drop your hands to their respective sides (Fig. 6).

As you raise your arms up, inhale. As you allow your arms to drop down, exhale. Be sure to focus your concentration on storing *chi,* or vital energy, in your abdomen when you reach figure five.

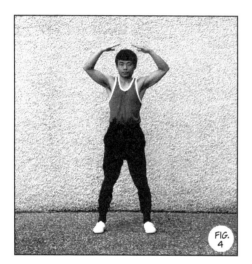
FIG. 4

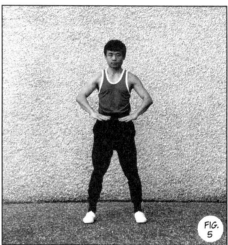
FIG. 5

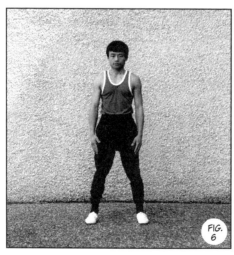
FIG. 6

Relax by Vibrating

Stand in a natural posture with your feet slightly apart. Now, using the flexing of your knees, bounce your body up and down 24 times (Figs. 7, 8), being sure to keep your feet flat on the ground as you do so. Next, twist your torso from side to side a number of times (Figs. 9, 10). After finishing the exercise, stand motionless for a few moments and breathe deeply. Finally, lightly massage your hands, head, and abdomen.

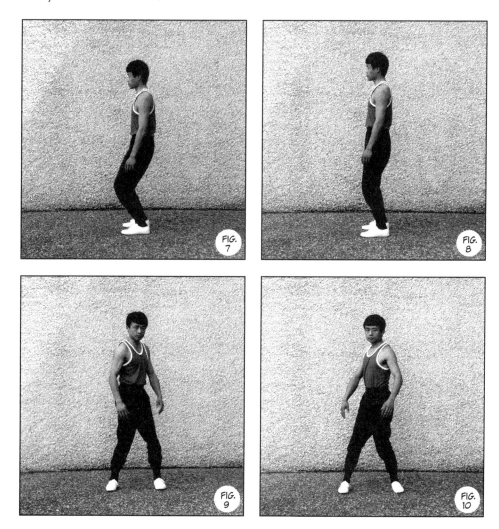

FIG. 7

FIG. 8

FIG. 9

FIG. 10

Set 9
DRY BATH EXERCISES

A dry bath is traditional Chinese technique for promoting the flow of vital energy, or *chi,* throughout the body. It is also particularly good for keeping skin healthy and youthful-looking. It can also serve as an effective method of relaxation.

The best time to practice the dry bath techniques is before bed or just after awakening in the morning. Apply light pressure to your skin during the dry bath. If you wish, you can use a soft cloth to rub your skin. Be sure to rub slowly and gently. When you massage your skin, use repetitions of 12 to 36 times.

Heaven's Drum
Stand in a relaxed, natural posture. Place your fingers on the back of your head with your palms over your ears (Fig. 1).

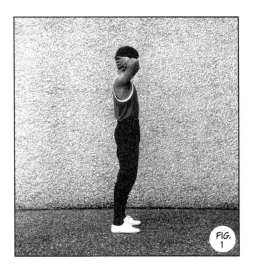

FIG. 1

Use your spread fingers to tap on the back of your head (Figs. 2, 3). Listen to the drumming sound. Breathe slowly and evenly.

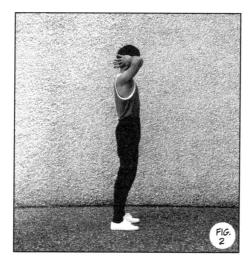

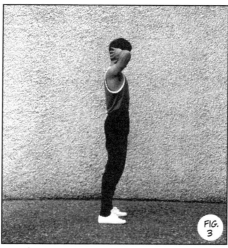

Face Bath

Begin with your hands resting on the lower part of your face (Fig. 4). Slide your hands up over your ears. Now slide your hands down to the starting position, but allow the middle fingers of either hand to glide over the side of your nose and the index finger of either hand to slide along the outer edge of your eyes. Rub back and forth in this manner.

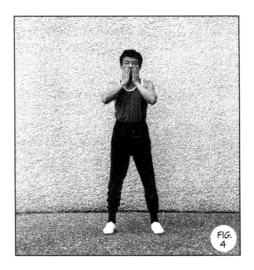

Now begin with your palms on the edge of your mouth and the first three fingers of either hand resting on the side of your nose. Slide your hands upward all the way into your hair, with your fingers acting as a comb (Fig. 5). Then slide your hands back over your head and along the back of your ears (Figs. 6, 7).

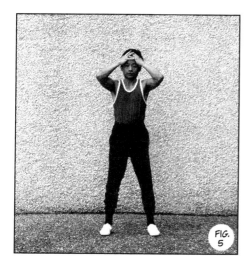

FIG. 5

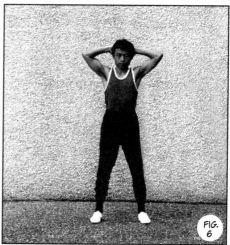

FIG. 6

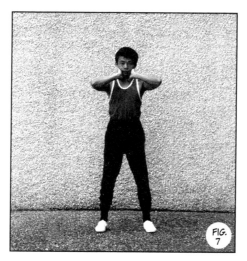

FIG. 7

Arm and Leg Bathing

Rub your left hand up and outside your right arm (Figs. 8, 9). Now rub your left hand inside and down your right arm (Figs. 10, 11).

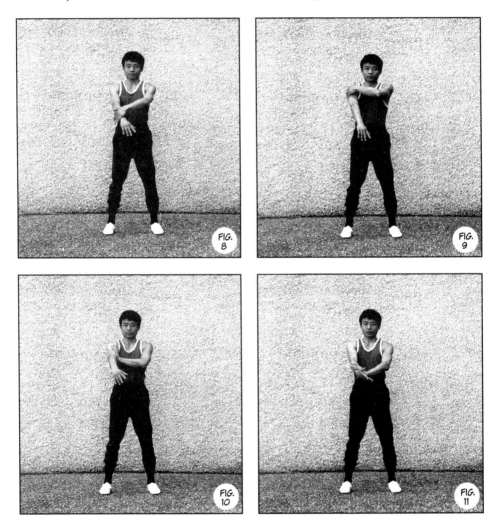

Repeat to the opposite side (Figs. 12–15).

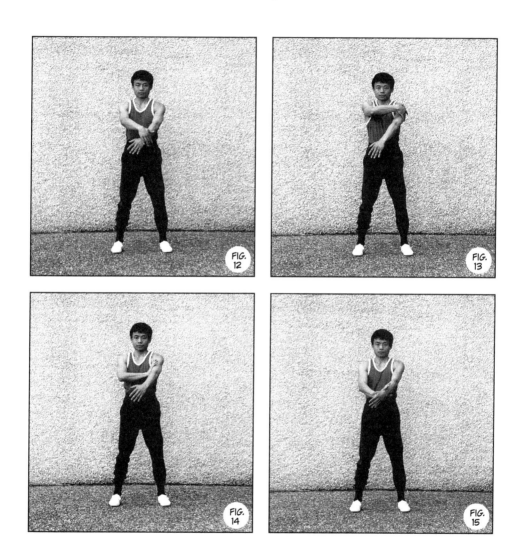

Rub your two hands from your rear down to your heels along the back of your legs. As you do so, allow your thumbs to slide down the side of your thighs (Figs. 16, 17). Now, rest your palms on the inside of your ankles and slide your hands up toward your groin (Figs. 18, 19).

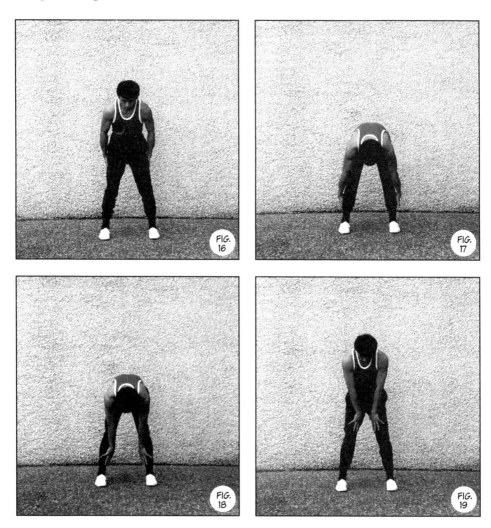

FIG. 16

FIG. 17

FIG. 18

FIG. 19

Belly Bathing

Place one hand on your stomach, with your fingers spread (Fig. 20). Rub your hand around your navel slowly with some pressure 10 to 20 times (Figs. 21–23).

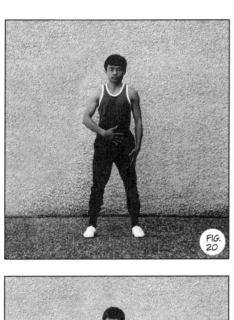

FIG. 20

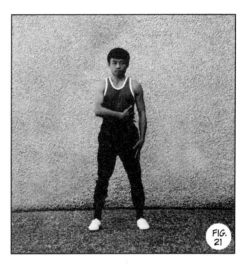

FIG. 21

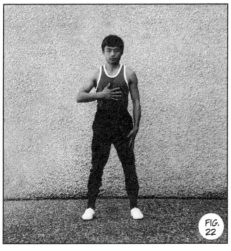

FIG. 22

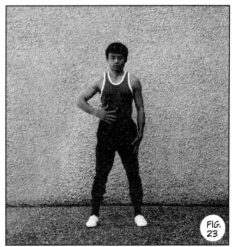

FIG. 23

After you have completed this set, switch to the other hand and perform the same sequence in the opposite direction (Figs. 24–27).

This exercise helps to alleviate digestive problems, but we suggest that pregnant women or people with stomach illnesses consult a doctor before doing it. As you rub your belly, concentrate on the space behind your navel and breathe slowly. Do not practice this exercise when you are hungry or right after a meal.

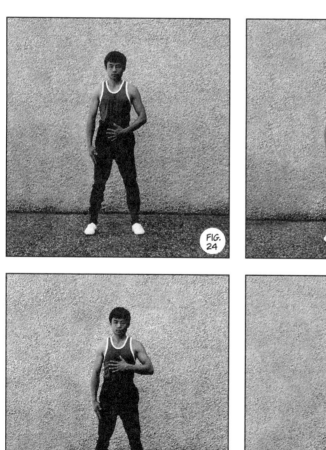

FIG. 24

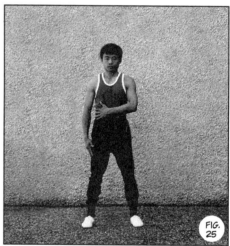

FIG. 25

FIG. 26

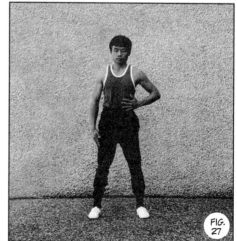

FIG. 27

PART TWO
ADVANCED EXERCISE SETS

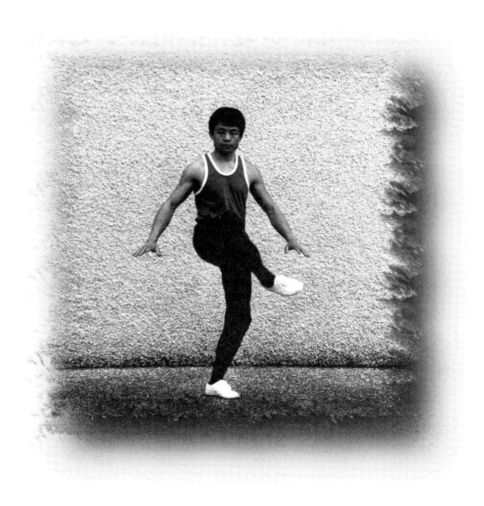

SET 10
TAI CHI CHUAN EXERCISES

Tai chi chuan is an ancient Chinese form of exercise and is also a martial art. It is designed to promote the production and flow of vital energy, and to make the body both stronger and more limber. Tai chi chuan is spoken of as being like "floating clouds and flowing streams," or like "pulling thread from a silk cocoon." Although it is a soft and slow form of exercise, it is also a martial art. This is why it is sometimes referred to as "a needle wrapped in cotton." Tai chi chuan is also said to help one concentrate power and energy inwardly, while maintaining a calm and peaceful outward appearance.

The correct way to master the art of tai chi chuan is to begin with a stationary pose and some simple repeated exercises. Some people might think it is a waste of time learning and practicing these basic exercises, but they actually serve to build a foundation from which you can more easily learn the more complicated techniques of tai chi chuan. These poses and exercises also help to develop one's vital energy, known as *chi*.

The first exercise we present, the standing pole, is essential for developing *chi*. The second exercise, sinking the *chi*, enables you to build a reservoir of *chi* and to master correct breathing. The rest of the exercises will build additional tai chi chuan skills.

As with the preceding exercises, when performing these tai chi chuan techniques you should remain focused on each movement rather than allowing yourself to daydream. Concentrate on keeping your breathing rhythmic and in harmony with your movements. Your body movements should be slow, soft, and graceful. Remain alert. Concentrate your spirit inwardly while appearing peaceful outwardly.

Standing Pole

Stand in a relaxed, straight posture with your feet parallel to one another and a shoulders-width apart (Fig. 1). Relax all of your joints, but do not intentionally bend any of your joints. Hold your head erect and relax your shoulders. Let your arms hang naturally with your palms facing your thighs. Draw in your chin, chest, belly, and buttocks to keep your backbone straight. Close your lips and allow the tip of your tongue to rest on the roof of your mouth behind your front teeth. Keep your eyes directed forward. Focus your attention on a spot about three inches behind your navel—this spot is known in Chinese as *dantien*. Breathe deeply, evenly, and slowly through your nose. Contract the lower abdomen while inhaling and expand it while exhaling.

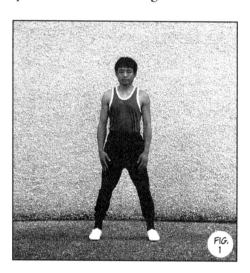

FIG. 1

Here are some tips that may help you visualize the proper posture for the standing pole exercise: Imagine that your head is suspended from the roof by a string that runs from the crown of your head, through your neck, along your spine to your tailbone. This will help you to keep your spine aligned correctly. With your mouth closed, touch your tongue to the roof of your mouth behind your front teeth as if you were going to make the sound "luh." Relax any tension in your chest and shoulders. Avoid allowing your stomach to protrude. Relax your fingers and knees. Concentrate on the *dantian*.

Stand in this posture, concentrating on your breathing and *dantian*, for five minutes a day. Increase your practice to twice a day, up to 15 or 20 minutes at a time. This exercise is beneficial for your entire body.

Sinking Chi into the Dantian

From a standing pole posture, raise your arms upward and slightly to the side with your palms facing downward. Imagine that your hands are resting on two balloons filled with helium that are slowly rising (Figs. 2, 3). As your hands reach shoulder level, bend your elbows to bring your hands in toward your body (Fig. 4). Now lower your hands down toward your navel with your thumbs pointing at one another (Fig. 5). This should feel like pushing a rubber ball into a pool of water.

Inhale as you raise your arms and exhale as you lower them. Remember to relax your shoulders and elbows as you raise your arms. When you lower your arms, try to feel the *chi* in your body fill the *dantian*. Repeat this exercise several times.

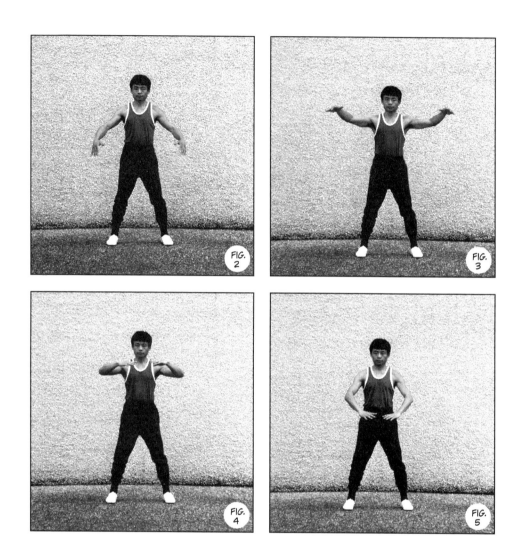

Stepping on Thin Ice

Extend your right foot, resting it slightly on the ball of the foot rather than on its heel. In this position, almost all of your weight should be on your left leg. Keep your hands out to their respective sides to help maintain balance (Fig. 6). From this posture, extend your right leg further, still keeping all of your weight on the left leg (Fig. 7). Imagine that you are about to step on a thin layer of ice. Slowly transfer about 70% of your weight onto your right leg (Fig. 8). Now lean back slightly and transfer most of your weight back onto your left leg (Fig. 9).

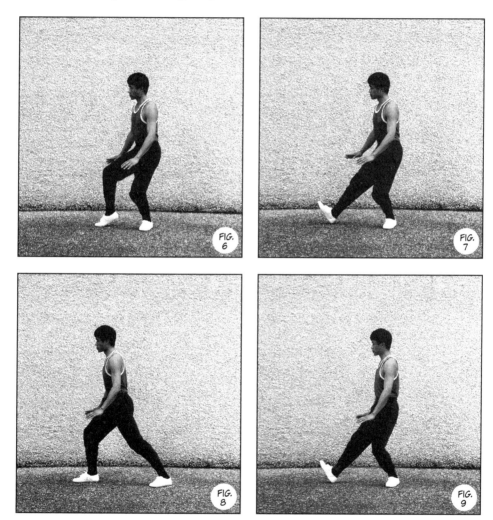

FIG. 6

FIG. 7

FIG. 8

FIG. 9

Turn your right foot out 45% to the right side, then pull your left leg forward as if withdrawing it from mud (Figs. 10–14). Now pull your left foot back, transferring your weight to your right foot (Fig. 15).

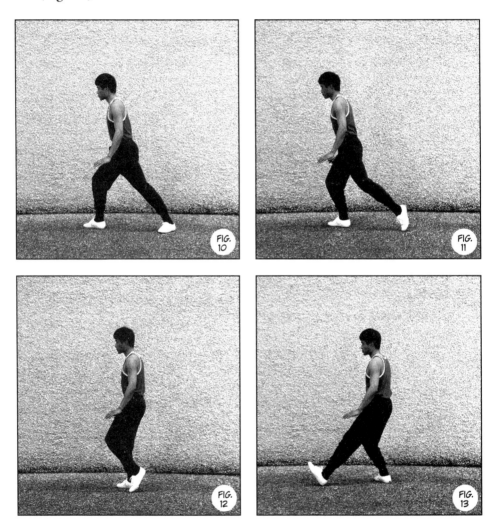

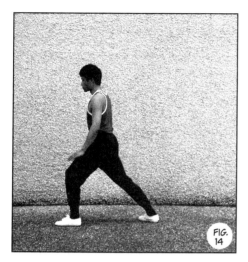

FIG.
14

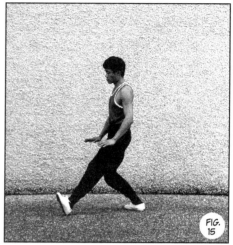

FIG.
15

Extend your left foot, resting it slightly on the ball of the foot rather than its heel, as you did previously with the right foot. Now step forward lightly with your left foot, as if treading on ice. Slowly transfer 70% of your weight onto your left leg (Fig. 16). Now lean back slightly and transfer most of your weight onto your right leg. Turn your left foot out 45% to the side, then pull your right leg forward as if withdrawing it from mud (Fig. 17). Continue.

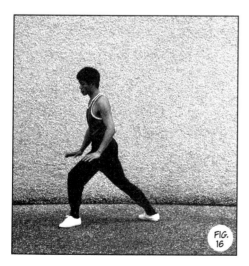

FIG.
16

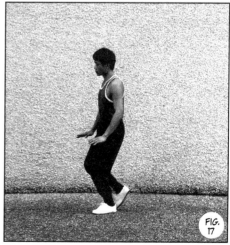

FIG.
17

Wave Hands Like Fish Tails

Stand in a relaxed posture with your feet slightly wider than the width of your shoulders. Wave your hands and arms back and forth in front of your chest in imitation of a fish tail in the water (Figs. 18–23). Imagine that you can feel the resistance of the water against your hands.

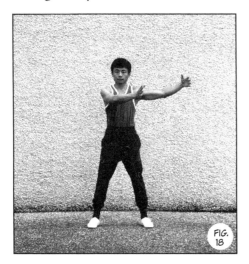
FIG. 18

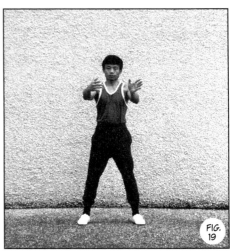
FIG. 19

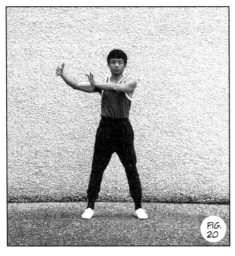
FIG. 20

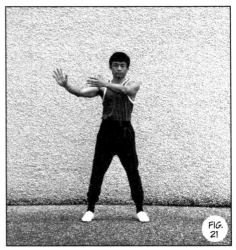
FIG. 21

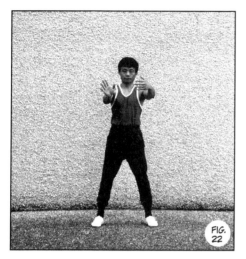

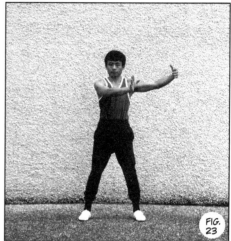

Now drop your hands to the front of your body (Fig. 24), and then wave your hands up and down, flexing your knees as you move them downward (Figs. 25–27).

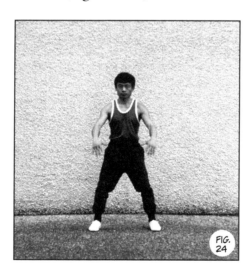

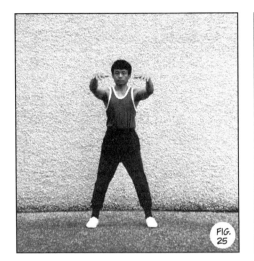

FIG. 25

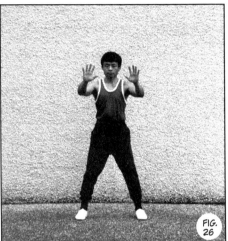

FIG. 26

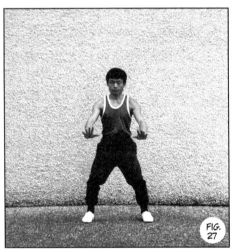

FIG. 27

Drawing a Circle

Tai chi chuan movements tend to be circular rather than linear. Not only are the techniques circular, but tai chi chuan practitioners try to keep their body gently curved during practice. This allows the *chi*, or vital energy, to flow through the body more easily.

The following circle drawing exercise will enable you to become familiar with the manner in which the hands are moved in tai chi chuan practice.

Begin in a relaxed posture with your right hand held in front of you with the palm facing to the left (Fig. 28). Now draw a counter-clockwise circle in front of your body, using your wrist as a focal point (Figs. 29–31). Pretend that your body is in a pool of water—imagine that you can feel the resistance of the water as your move your arm in a circle. Allow your hand to bend because of the resistance of the water. You can make a circle in either a clockwise or counterclockwise direction. Switch to the other arm.

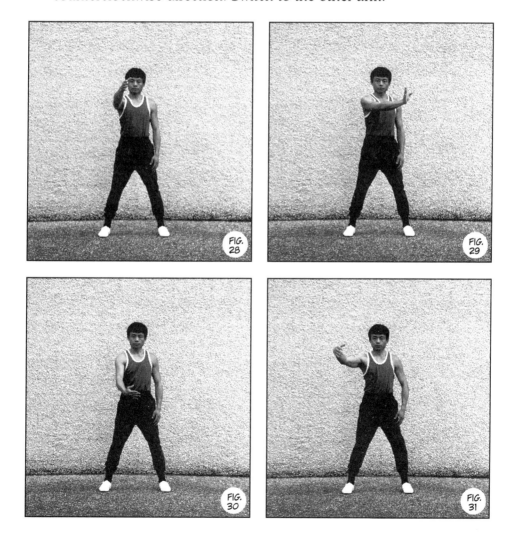

FIG. 28

FIG. 29

FIG. 30

FIG. 31

Now try the exercise with two arms. Begin with both arms held in front of you with palms facing (Fig. 32). Bring both arms together as you begin drawing the circle (Fig. 33). Make a counter-clockwise circle with your right arm and a clockwise circle with your left arm (Figs. 34, 35).

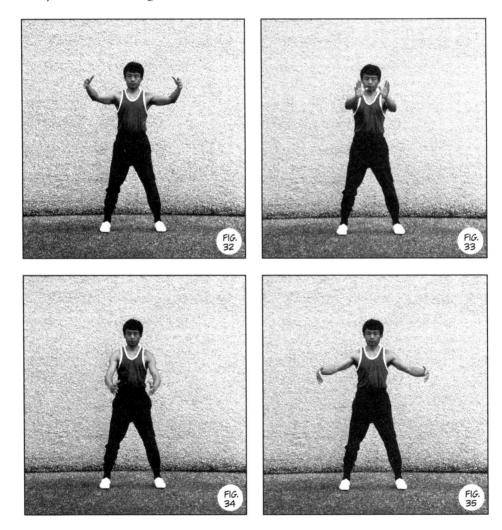

FIG. 32

FIG. 33

FIG. 34

FIG. 35

You can also rotate both arms in the same direction, but stagger the movements so that one hand is up while the other is down (Figs. 36–39).

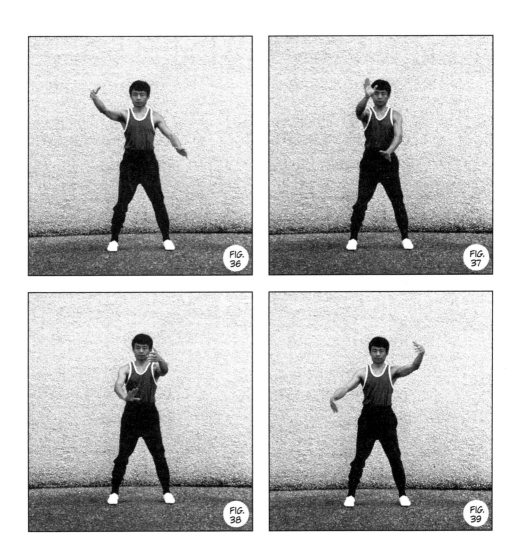

Hanging Leg

Stand on your left leg with your hands held out at waist level to their respective sides (Fig. 40). Your right knee should be held at waist level. Now, using your knee as a fulcrum, rotate your foot in a circular direction (Figs. 41–43).

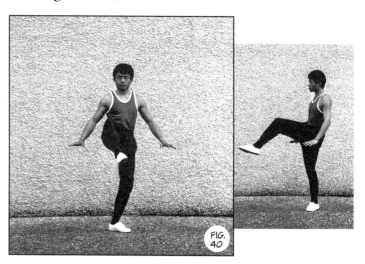

FIG. 40

This exercise will increase your ability to maintain balance, which is important when kicking or stepping toward an opponent in self-defense. You can either bend or straighten the standing leg and you can either draw a smaller or larger circle with your hanging leg.

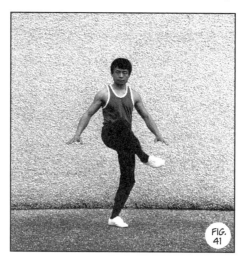

FIG. 41

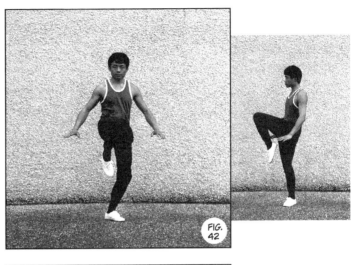

FIG. 42

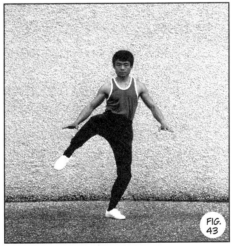

FIG. 43

Pushing Against Waves

Stand in a relaxed posture. Imagine you are standing up to your chest in the ocean with your back to the beach. Extend your arms toward the water with palms down (Fig. 44). Pretend that a wave washes over you, pushing your hands back toward your chest with palms facing forward (Fig. 45). Now push forward against the waves (Figs. 46, 47). Inhale as you retract your hands and exhale as you push forward.

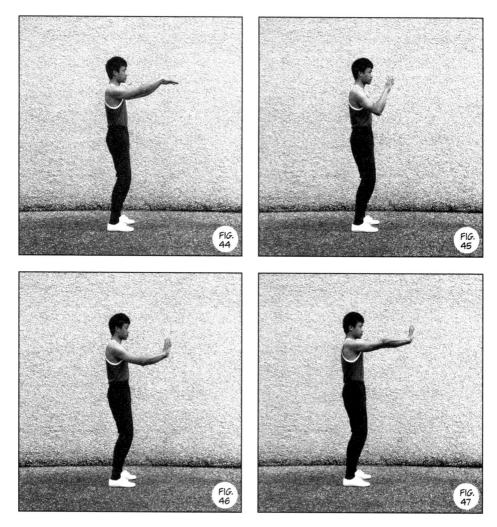

Waist and Step Turning

Begin with your hands on your hips and your feet slightly wider than shoulders-width (Fig. 48). Step out to the right with your right foot (Fig. 49). Transfer 70% of your weight onto your left leg, then turn your torso to the right (Fig. 50). Transfer 70% of your weight onto your right leg as you bend your right knee and move your torso forward (Fig. 51).

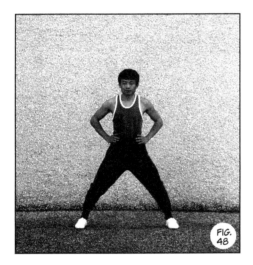

FIG. 48

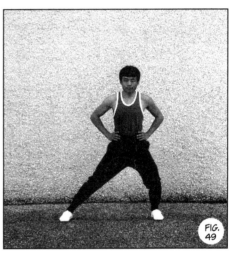

FIG. 49

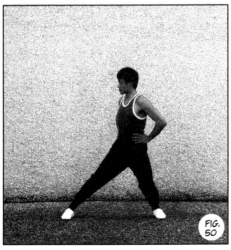

FIG. 50

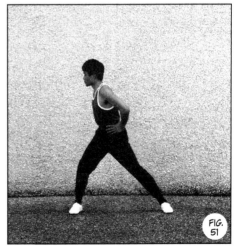

FIG. 51

While practicing, you should be aware that your legs are the base and your waist is the axis. The whole body is in constant motion throughout the exercise. Breathe in while turning your trunk and breathe out while moving your weight.

Repeat in the opposite direction (Figs. 52–55).

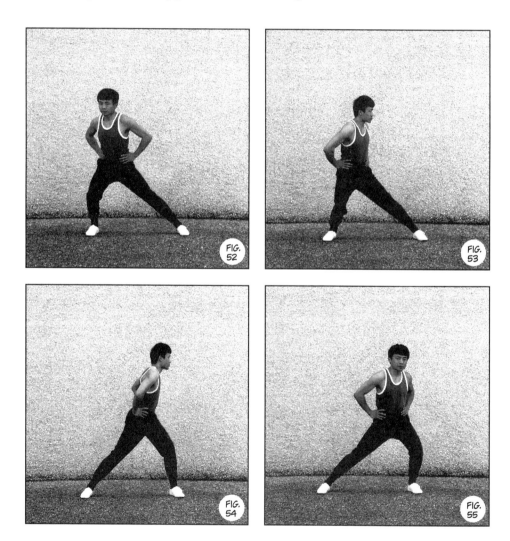

Working the Millstone

Step forward with your right leg. Keep your right knee bent and your left leg straight. Extend your hands in front of you with the palms facing down (Fig. 56). Increasingly shift your weight onto your back leg as you make a counterclockwise circle parallel to the ground with your hands (Figs. 57, 58).

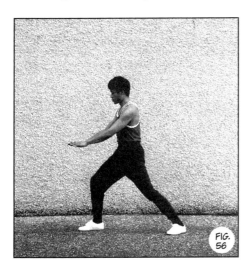

FIG. 56

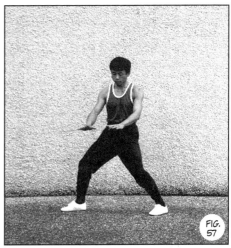

FIG. 57

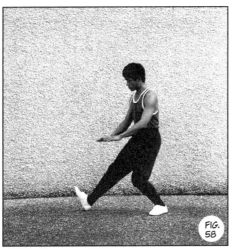

FIG. 58

As you finish the circle, transfer your weight back onto your front leg (Figs. 59, 60). Repeat to the opposite side (Figs. 61–64).

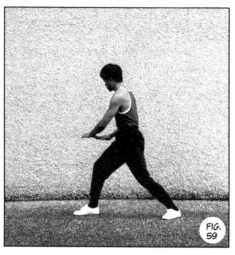

FIG. 59

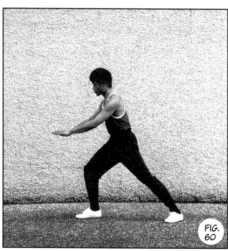

FIG. 60

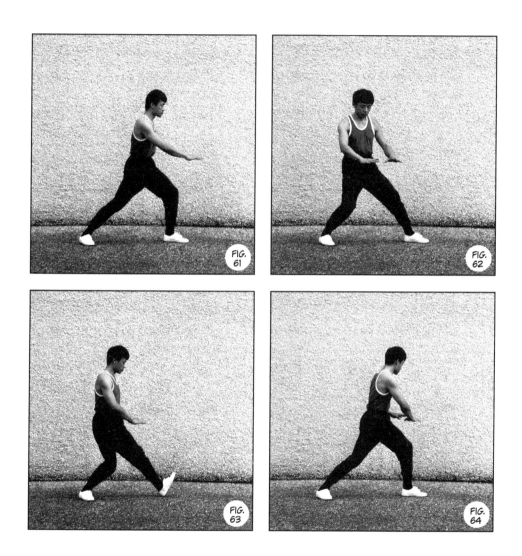

FIG. 61

FIG. 62

FIG. 63

FIG. 64

Wave Hands Like Clouds

This is a comprehensive exercise that combines all the skills developed in the previous exercises. Begin with your torso facing forward and your knees slightly bent. Place your right hand in front of your chin with the palm toward your face and your left hand in front of your navel with the palm directed downward (Fig. 65). Shift your weight slightly to the right, turn your torso to the right, and swing your arms to the right (Figs. 66, 67).

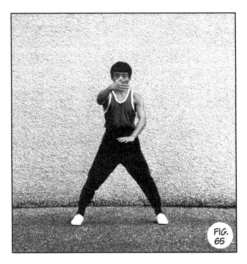

FIG. 65

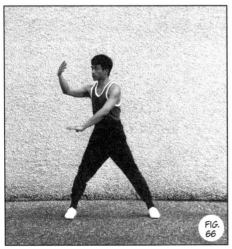

FIG. 66

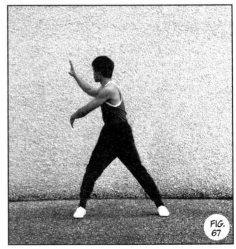

FIG. 67

Lift your left hand to chest level while lowering your right hand (Fig. 68). Shift your weight back to the left as you turn in that direction (Figs. 69–71).

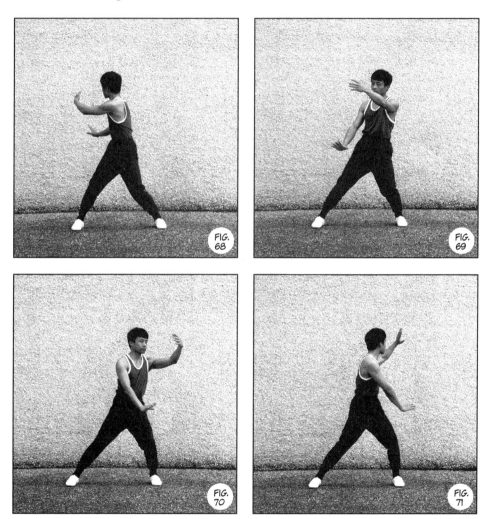

FIG. 68

FIG. 69

FIG. 70

FIG. 71

Now raise your right hand and lower your left hand in preparation for turning back to the right (Fig. 72).

As you switch the position of your hands, inhale. Keep your shoulders relaxed as you wave your arms. Keep your fingers curled slightly inward in a relaxed position.

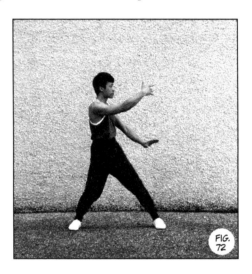

FIG. 72

SET 11
SINEW TRANSFORMING EXERCISES

According to legend, a famous Buddhist monk by the name of Damo, or Bodhidharma, invented the *yi jin jing*, or "sinew transforming exercise," about 1,500 years ago. Damo, who was the founder of the Zen school of Buddhism (also known as Ch'an in Chinese), devised this exercise to improve the health of Buddhist monks who spent almost all of their time sitting in quiet meditation. This exercise routine later became a basic form of training for the famous Shaolin monks.

The traditional routine contains 12 separate exercises. Although it is time consuming, it is relatively easy to learn compared to the various other internal exercise, or *qigong* routines that are in current use among practitioners of the Chinese martial arts. Today, the sinew transforming exercise is still learned as a fundamental part of Chinese martial training, but is also useful for maintaining health and preventing illness.

Practice this routine in a quiet place that has a good supply of fresh air (but no strong wind). Wear loose and comfortable clothing.

Please note that when performing these exercises, you should move slowly and softly. Relax your body and mind. Breathe slowly and deeply through your nose. Concentrate on the *dantian*.

Preparatory Pose

Stand erect and relaxed with your feet parallel to one another about a shoulder's width apart. Your back should be straight and your hands should hang at your sides. Close your lips and allow the tip of your tongue to rest on the roof of your mouth behind your front teeth. Breathe evenly and slowly through your nose. Look forward, but concentrate your attention on your *dantian* (Fig. 1).

As with the standing pole, this is a beginning posture that will help you to clear your mind and relax your body.

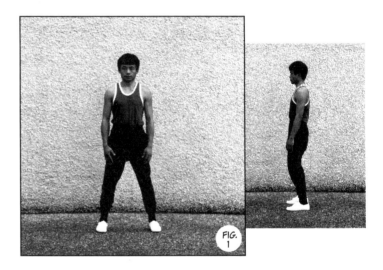

FIG.
1

Pressed Palms Pose

From the previous pose, raise your arms to chest level with your palms facing downward, inhaling as you do so (Fig. 2). Bring your palms together in front of your chest, exhaling as you do so (Figs. 3, 4). Your fingers should point toward your throat. Keep your fingertips and the heels of your hands together, while allowing the center of your palms to arch slightly. Hold this pose for five to 15 minutes.

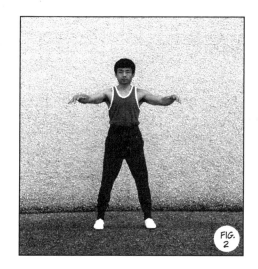

FIG. 2

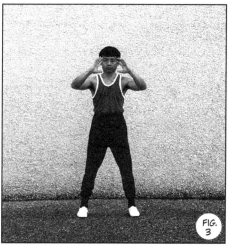

FIG. 3

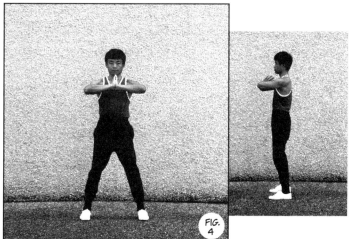

FIG. 4

Extended Arms Pose

Beginning from the pressed palms pose, lower your hands to your navel, with palms downward, exhaling as you do so (Fig. 5). Then raise your arms sideways to shoulder level, inhaling as you do so (Figs. 6, 7). As you raise your arms, lift your heels off the ground. Stretch your arms. Focus on the palms of your hands and the arches of your feet. These are *chi* gates known in acupuncture as *laogong* and *yongquan*.

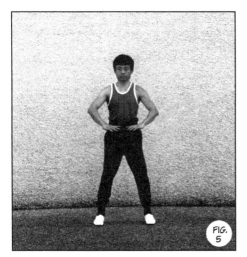

FIG. 5

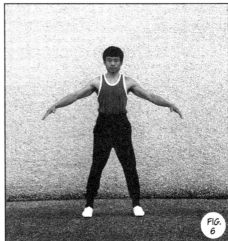

FIG. 6

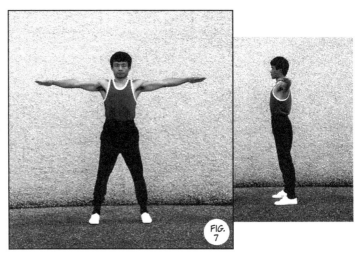

FIG. 7

Propping Up the Sky

Beginning from the previous pose, raise your arms above your head until your palms face one another with your fingers pointing upward (Figs. 8, 9).

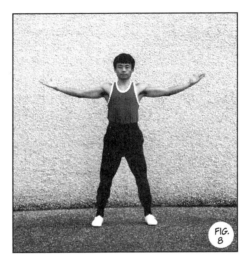

FIG. 8

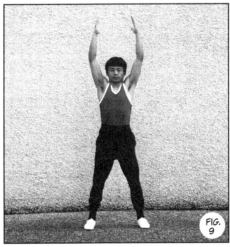

FIG. 9

Then turn your hands so that your palms face upward. Look straight up between your hands and stretch your arms a little (Fig. 10). Inhale as you perform the above motion. Keep your backbone straight and relaxed. Breathe gently through your nose. Hold this position as long as you can. Then lower your arms to return to the basic posture. Relax.

When inhaling, focus on the centers of your palms. As you drop your arms down, exhale and focus on the arches of your feet.

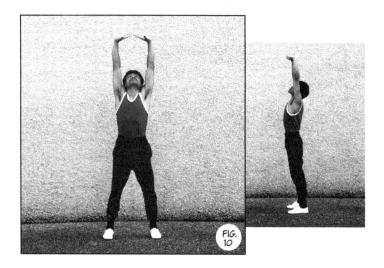

FIG.
10

Catching a Star

Beginning in the basic posture, lift your left arm to the side with the palm up and place your right hand behind your back, inhaling as you do so (Fig. 11). Raise your left arm up over your head and stretch the arm with the palm of your hand facing toward the sky (Fig. 12).

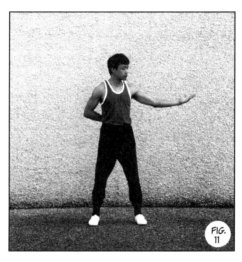

FIG. 11

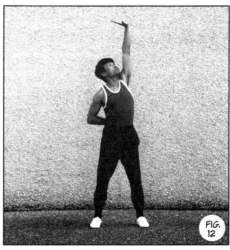

FIG. 12

Your weight should shift slightly onto your right leg and your body should turn to the left. Bend your right knee slightly and turn your left palm toward your face, exhaling as you do so (Fig. 13). Hold this pose. Repeat on the opposite side (Fig. 14). Return to the basic posture.

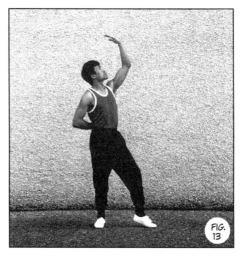

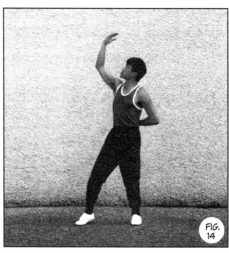

Pulling the Bull's Tail

Spread your feet slightly (Fig. 15). Extend your left leg to the left side. Curl your left arm with your hand in a fist. Hold your right arm behind you with the hand in a fist (Fig. 16). Imagine pulling a weight backward with your left arm, bending backward and exhaling as you do so (Fig. 17). Now pull with your right arm and lean forward. Repeat on the opposite side (Fig. 18). When you pull with the front arm, inhale. When you pull with the back arm, exhale. Return to the basic posture.

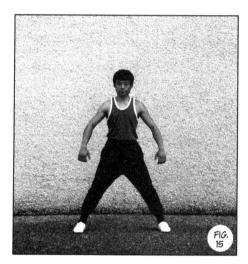

FIG. 15

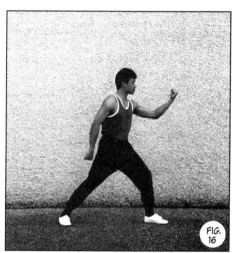

FIG. 16

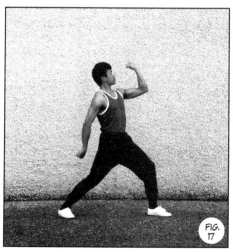

FIG. 17

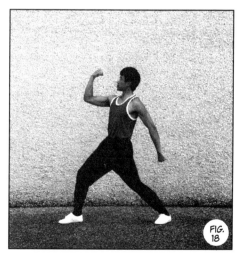

FIG. 18

Forward Push

Lift your arms to shoulder level, inhaling as you do so (Fig. 19). Now push forward with the palms of your hands, exhaling as you do so (Figs. 20, 21). Retract your hands to your chest as you inhale. Push forward again. Repeat this exercise seven times. Return to the basic posture.

In the beginning, push forward softly, but then begin to use more force. At the end, imagine pushing an enormous weight. At the point of extension, spread your fingers and try to push your palms forward as much as possible.

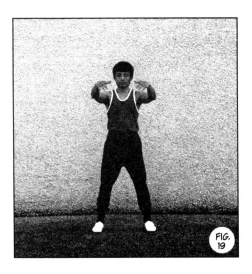

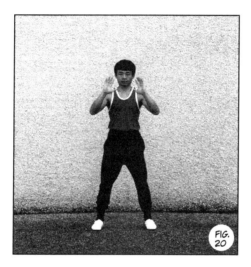

FIG. 20

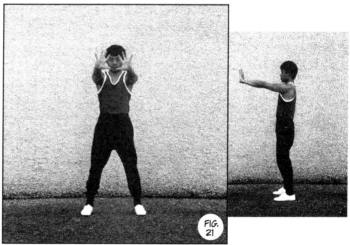

FIG. 21

Drawing the Sword

Lift your right arm to your chest with the palm of your hand facing inward. Lift your left hand so that the back of the hand rests on your lower back (Fig. 22). Continue to lift your right hand over your head. Rest the palm of your right hand against the back of your head (Fig. 23).

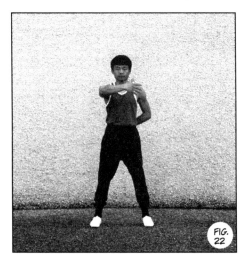

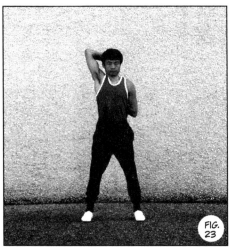

Grasp your left ear with your index and middle finger, then turn your waist and head to the left and look backward (Fig. 24). Inhale as you perform the twisting motion. Hold this pose. Then lower your hands and repeat on the opposite side (Fig. 25). Return to the basic posture.

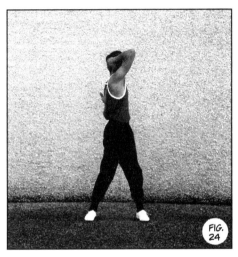

FIG. 24

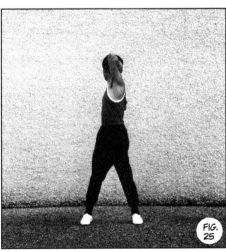

FIG. 25

Lowering Toward the Ground

Inhale and lift your arms to shoulder level with the palms of your hands facing upward. Turn your hands so that your palms face downward, then lower your arms as you begin to sink down into a squat (Fig. 26). Continue to lower your arms as you sink down, exhaling as you do so (Fig. 27).

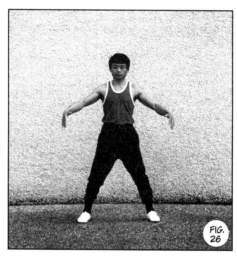

FIG. 26

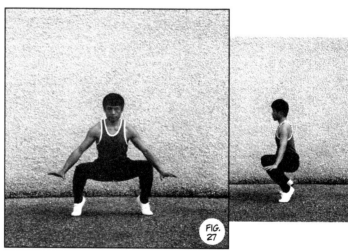

FIG. 27

Lift your heels off the ground as you squat. Hold this pose. Then turn your palms upward and lift your arms up to shoulder level as you rise up (Fig. 28). Swing your hands inward and press your palms together. Then return to the basic posture.

Imagine that you are pressing two balloons into a pool of water while squatting, and lifting some heavy objects while standing up.

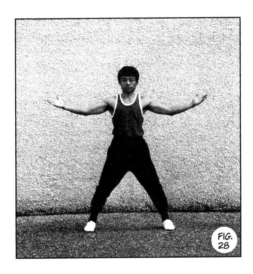

FIG. 28

Extending the Claw

Lift your hands to your waist. Extend your left arm to its side with the palm of your hand facing upward (Fig. 29). In an arc, lift your left arm up and over your head as you inhale (Fig. 30). At the end of the movement, your left arm should be nearly touching your left ear and the palm of your hand should face downward. Hold this pose.

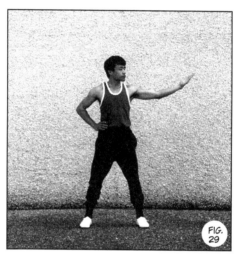

FIG. 29

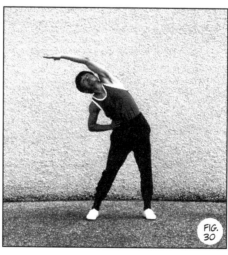

FIG. 30

Then lower your left hand, turning your wrist so that the palm of your hand faces upward as you squat down (Fig. 31). Exhale as you squat. Continue the circular motion of your arm by bringing your left hand back to your waist as you rise up to a standing position. Repeat on the opposite side (Fig. 32).

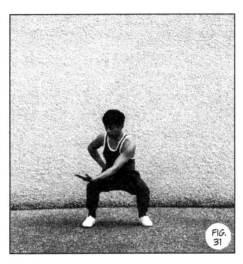

FIG. 31

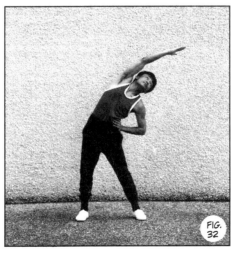

FIG. 32

Tiger Pose

Turn to the left and step forward with your left leg, as shown (Fig. 33). As you turn, raise your hands to your waist with your palms facing upward. Push your arms forward with your hands in a tiger claw position (Fig. 34). Swing your arms and torso down and touch your fingertips by your front foot. As you do so, exhale and make a sound like "ha." Inhale as you lift your head to look forward (Fig. 35). Hold this pose.

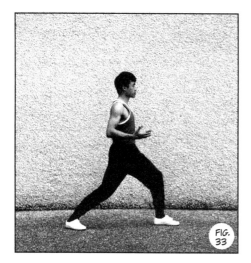
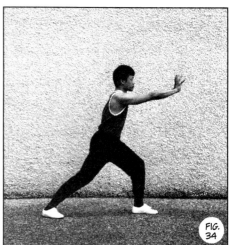
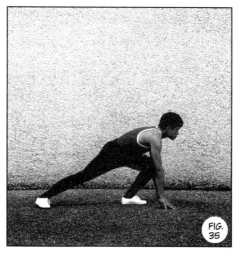

Repeat on the opposite side (Fig. 36).

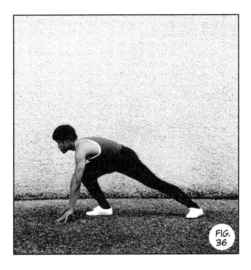

Return to the basic posture.

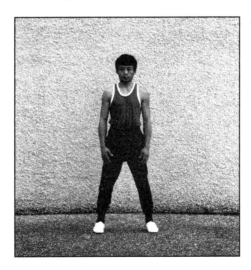

Bang the Drum

Raise your arms and bend your elbows to rest your hands against the back of your head (Figs. 37, 38). Inhale as you make this movement. Slide your hands to cover your ears with your palms as you bend over (Fig. 39). Exhale as you bend. Drum on the back of your head with your fingertips. Return to the basic posture.

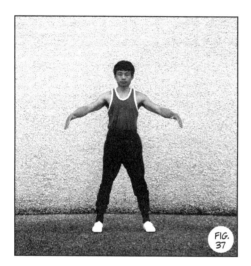

FIG. 37

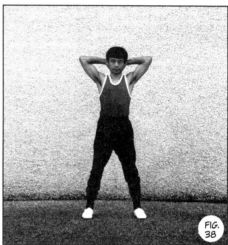

FIG. 38

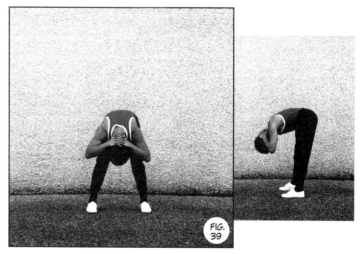

FIG. 39

Pushing Down Pose

Lift your hands to chest level with your palms pointing downward, inhaling as you do so (Fig. 40). Now push your hands straight down and bend at the waist, exhaling as you do so (Fig. 41). If you prefer, you can lock your fingers together as you stretch (Fig. 42). Hold this position. Do not bend your knees. Return to the basic posture.

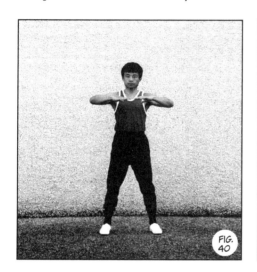

FIG. 40

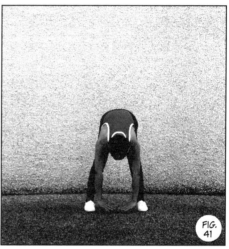

FIG. 41

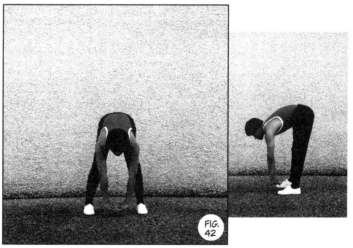

FIG. 42

The Closing Form

Stand in the preparatory pose for a moment. Then lift your heels off the ground and, flexing your knees, bounce up and down on your feet 21 times (Figs. 43, 44). Allow your body to bounce in a relaxed manner. This is known as jolting.

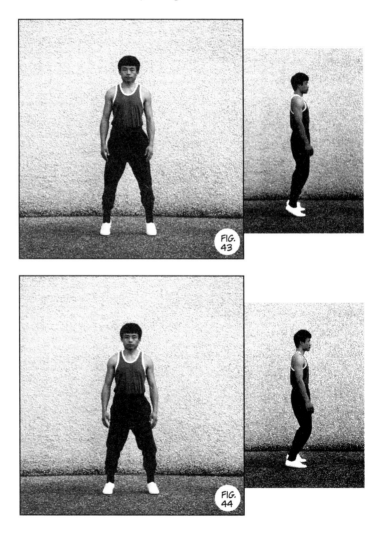

FIG. 43

FIG. 44

Now lift your right arm and shake it out to the right side as if it were a garden hose. As you allow your right arm to drop down, repeat this motion with your left arm (Figs. 45–50). This is known as spreading arms. Shake each arm about seven times, then stand still for a moment, breathing deeply. Finally, lightly massage your hands, head, and abdomen.

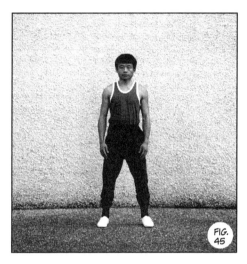

FIG. 45

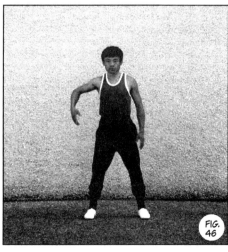

FIG. 46

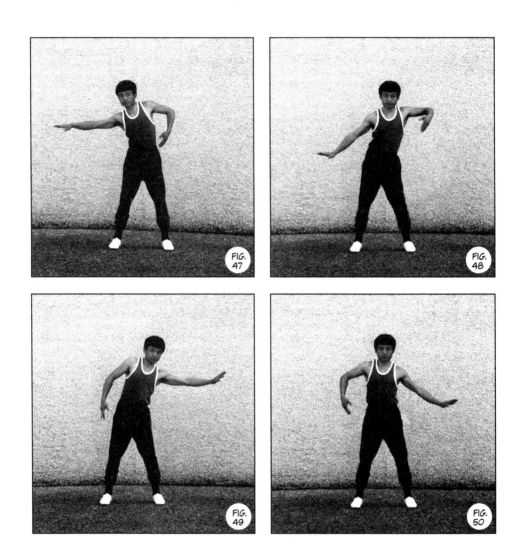